Karola Muther

The nursing consultationin the oncological setting

Karola Muther

The nursing consultationin the oncological setting

Monograph

ScienciaScripts

Imprint
Any brand names and product names mentioned in this book are subject to trademark, brand or patent protection and are trademarks or registered trademarks of their respective holders. The use of brand names, product names, common names, trade names, product descriptions etc. even without a particular marking in this work is in no way to be construed to mean that such names may be regarded as unrestricted in respect of trademark and brand protection legislation and could thus be used by anyone.

Cover image: www.ingimage.com

This book is a translation from the original published under ISBN 978-3-639-46628-7.

Publisher:
Sciencia Scripts
is a trademark of
Dodo Books Indian Ocean Ltd. and OmniScriptum S.R.L publishing group

120 High Road, East Finchley, London, N2 9ED, United Kingdom
Str. Armeneasca 28/1, office 1, Chisinau MD-2012, Republic of Moldova, Europe
Printed at: see last page
ISBN: 978-620-5-67543-4

Contents

ACKNOWLEDGMENTS 2

BRIEF 3

ABSTRACT 4

1 Introduction 5

2 Theoretical part 10

3 Empirical part 37

4 Presentation of the results 64

5 Summary and résumé 78

6 Outlook and Limitation 82

BIBLIOGRAPHY 84

ANNEX 90

THANKS

My special thanks go to my work colleagues, my family and especially to my husband Dieter, who accompanied and supported me throughout my studies.

Furthermore, I would like to thank my nursing service management and division management, who gave me enough freedom to write my Master's thesis.

I would also like to thank my supervisor, Mr. Jonathan Jancsary, MA, BA for his motivation and appreciation during my Master's thesis preparation.

Your support has contributed significantly to the success of my study.

Karola Muther

BRIEF

Background

The nursing consultation in the oncological setting in a primary care hospital is perceived as a special challenge by the staff of the higher service for health care and nursing. Above all, it involves being able to engage in conversations with patients and their relatives, which are characterised by complex questions. Nurses in the oncology setting are therefore required to engage in conversation and communication in order to develop a deeper understanding of counselling.

Destination

The aim of this study is to experience, identify and understand fundamental issues that arise in the context of a nursing counselling session in the oncology setting, as well as a focus on difficulties, obstacles and the unexpected in the context of a counselling session.

Methodology

The research methodology of grounded theory is selected for the present work.

Results/Conclusion

Communication in the form of counselling is carried out with a high degree of professionalism by the staff of the higher service for health care and nursing, but they lack awareness of their interactive work. This means for the company that the specific professionalism of interactive work must be demanded and therefore education, training and further education in the field of nursing must be expanded.

Keywords

Oncological setting, nursing counselling, counselling skills, interactive communication

ABSTRACT

Background

Nursing consultation within an oncological setting in a primary health care centre above all includes being able to get involved into conversation, marked by complex questions, with the patients and their family members. Therefore, nurses in an oncological setting are asked to pay attention to conversation techniques and communication. As a result, a more profound understanding of nursing consultation can be developed.

Objective

The objective of this study is to discover, identify and understand general topics that emerge in the context of a nursing consultation within an oncological setting, as well as to focus on difficulties, obstacles and unexpected issues that may arise within the context of consultations.

Methodology

For the present study, the research methodology "Grounded Theory" has been chosen.

Results/conclusion

Communication in terms of consultation is provided by the employees of the "Gehobener Dienst fur Gesundheits- und Krankenpflege" (Advanced Service for Health and Nursing Care) with a high level of professionality. There is, however, a lack of awareness of their interactive work. For the company this entails that the specific professionality of interactive work must be facilitated. Therefore, formations, trainings and further education in the nursing sector must be expanded.

Keywords

Oncological setting, nursing consultation, consultation competences, interactive communication.

1 Introduction

The topic of "counselling" is becoming increasingly important in professional care. In everyday nursing care, however, counselling often accompanies action. The value of communicative nursing work tends to fade into the background. Nurses often have a guilty conscience when they talk too long with patients and their relatives. The expectations and previous experiences as well as the emotional state of patients and their relatives make communication difficult in the oncological setting. The demand for communication skills in oncological care could reduce anxiety during the disease process (cf. Kennedy, 2005).

The author of this research has therefore looked at the counselling conversation of oncology patients and their relatives from the nurses' point of view, so that it can be recorded that the complexity of conversations in the oncology setting consists not only of specific professional knowledge, but above all of psychological, social and pastoral content. This, in turn, shows that nurses in the oncology setting are required to engage in conversation and, by extension, counselling.

1.1 Problem

Cancer diseases are systemic diseases that require a holistic, multidisciplinary and long-term treatment of the affected patients. Employees of the senior health and nursing service must therefore face new challenges because, on the one hand, patients with these diseases require intensive care and support and, on the other hand, the next of kin need professional support. The special setting of an oncology department places high demands on the staff of the higher service of health care and nursing. Complex work processes, but also the everyday confrontation with seriously ill patients and their emotional starting position are aspects that need to be taken into account. Communicating the necessary treatment and care measures in an understandable and up-to-date manner is an essential part of their work (Bachmann-Mettler, 2007: 356).

In professional interactions with people, awareness is necessary of why something is said, what technique is used, but also why something is not said. It requires time, practice and reflection on the part of the carer. If done well or poorly, conversational interactions can be remembered by patients and their families as well as by the nurses themselves (cf. Radziewicz & Baile, 2001; Virani, Malloy, Ferrell & Kelly, 2008).

Counselling discussions in care do not have a clearly defined counselling setting and therefore counselling in everyday care often takes place during care activities. Hummel-Gaatz and Doll 2006 define counselling as follows:

"Counselling is a relational process between carers or their caregivers (family and/or friends) with the aim of supporting them in coping with illness and crisis. This is done by supporting them in coping with problems, supporting them in finding decisions, demanding, discovering and maintaining resources, supporting them in dealing with changed life circumstances and the resulting consequences" (Hummel-Gaatz, Doll 2006: 16).

The oncological counselling interview in a primary care hospital in Vorarlberg is perceived as a special challenge by the staff of the higher service for health care and nursing. Above all, it involves being able to spontaneously engage in conversations with patients and their relatives, characterised by complex questions. In their everyday professional life, however, nurses are often overwhelmed in their role as mediator, contact person and confidant, and are also exhausted, helpless and at a loss. Especially after the doctor has given bad news, the nurses are the first contact person for the patients and their relatives. The nurses also describe communication with demanding relatives as stressful and difficult. The work activities of the staff in the higher service for health care and nursing in this oncology department in a basic care hospital in Vorarlberg differ from the other disciplines in that there is an increased need for communication and cooperation between the nursing staff, doctors, patients and their relatives. Nurses in oncology are therefore called upon to engage in conversation and communication so that a deeper understanding of counselling can develop as a result.

The author of this Master's thesis wanted to reflect on the challenges that arise in the oncology department of a primary care hospital in Vorarlberg for the senior nursing staff (specifically in the oncology counselling interview) and to provide suggestions for improvement.

1.2 Objective

The aim of this research work is to record the current situation in a primary care hospital in Vorarlberg, how staff members of the higher service for health care and nursing perceive their role as a confidant and mediator in the oncological counselling interview. The study aims to show the challenges during a consultation from the staff's point of view, so that supportive measures can be offered in the future.

A clear non-objective is to record the frequency of stresses and strains of the staff of the higher service for health care and nursing in the oncological setting.

Another non-objective is to assess the needs of relatives of patients with cancer in the oncology setting.

1.3 Research question

The oncological counselling interview in a primary care hospital in Vorarlberg is perceived as a special challenge by the staff of the higher service for health care and nursing. Above all, it involves being able to spontaneously engage in conversations characterised by complex questions with patients and their relatives. In their everyday professional life, however, nurses are often overwhelmed in their role as mediator, contact person and confidant, and are also exhausted, helpless and at a loss. In this research work, the author therefore deals with the following central question and concretising sub-questions:

How do staff members of the higher service for health care and nursing experience the nursing counselling interview with patients and their relatives in the oncological setting of a primary care hospital in Vorarlberg?

- How do nurses distinguish themselves in the nursing counselling interview?
- What framework conditions are necessary for professional nursing counselling to be carried out?
- What is the relationship of the nurses to the patients and their relatives?
- What role does the doctor/nurse relationship play?
- What previous knowledge and experience do nurses have in nursing counselling?

1.4 Methodology

For the present work, the research methodology of grounded theory is selected. Grounded theory is a set of procedures designed to lead to the discovery of theoretical data and used for the ultimate purpose of theory building on the basis of empirical data (cf. Glaser, Straus, 1967).

Grounded theory is a qualitative research method with the aim of indicating systematic ways of deriving theories from field data and thus strategically demanding the anchoring of research in the field (cf. Lueger, 2009).

Grounded theory is particularly suitable for the investigation of phenomena where personal experience is important. The research question should provide the necessary flexibility and freedom to investigate a phenomenon in depth. Not all concepts related to the phenomenon being researched are found and identified (Strauss, Corbin, 1996: 22).

The literature search was conducted in the library of the University of Vienna and in scientific, social science and psychological databases for medicine and health sciences EBSCO Cinahl, Evidence Based Medicine with Reviews, Medline and Ovid. For an extensive literature search, key words, generic and subordinate terms, core terms, synonyms, inclusion and exclusion criteria as well as English translations using "linguee" were used in order not to overlook any important search terms during the literature search. The Boolean operators AND and OR were used to combine search terms. Further research was conducted in the journals and e-journals Pflege, Padua, EvidenceBased Nursing and Journal of Advanced Nursing.

The study consists of narrative interviews, which are conducted face-to-face with six staff members of the senior health and nursing service in the oncology setting in a primary care hospital in Vorarlberg. The test persons are asked to report on certain situations and how they experience them. The course of the interview was to be flexible in order to ensure an unhindered flow of speech.

Data evaluation is a continuous comparison in a three-step coding process and a circular process involving the linking of data collection and evaluation. The first step (open coding) consists of "breaking down" the data. This means that texts are divided into units of analysis and discovered phenomena are labelled with codes, bundled and classified into superordinate categories. The second step (axial coding) involves the search for possible empirical connections between the categories. The third step (selective coding) consists of identifying the core categories. Reflection is an important good criterion throughout the research process and helps to open the view, the possibilities of perception and action for new and foreign things. Ongoing self-reflection and reflection on topics, as well as one's own professional experience, are prerequisites in dealing with the research material (cf. Breuer et al., 2009: 59f).

The topic of this research meets the characteristics and requirements and justifies the application of Grounded Theory. The data is processed in a detailed, intensive and systematic analysis that leads to the development of concepts that characterise, interpret and explain the central phanomena.

1.5 Structure of the work

The first chapter of this research paper deals with the problem, the objective, the research question and the methodology of data collection and analysis and the procedure of the work. Chapter two provides an overview of the current state of research. Here, the basics of counselling concepts, specifically the concept of counselling in care, legal foundations in counselling as well as the counselling process in care and the goal of counselling are explained. This is followed by the basics of communicative competences, which describe client-centred conversation according to Carl R. Rogers and human communication according to Paul Watzlawick in more detail. An introduction to verbal, non-verbal and para-verbal communication is also given. Counselling skills in nursing are the prerequisite for professional counselling. The oncological counselling interview is described on the basis of the phases of a cancer disease, so that it becomes clear which different types of language and counselling are used. Finally, the structure and the course of an oncological counselling interview are discussed.

In chapter three, the current research follows. A qualitative research approach is chosen. The research question relates to the nature of experiences and the experience of dealing with oncology patients and their relatives. Experiences are to be documented and analysed through an intensive dialogue with senior health and nursing staff in the oncology setting. The data collection method is based on open-ended interviews with six staff members of the senior health and nursing service of an oncology department of a primary care hospital in Vorarlberg. The aim of this work is therefore not to determine, with the help of a quantitative analysis, how frequently various stresses occur in oncology departments, but how nurses perceive, talk about and deal with these challenges in the oncology counselling interview. Chapter four presents the results of the interviews. The data is analysed using grounded theory. In chapter five there is a discussion and comparison of the research question with the theory. In chapter six there is a summary and résumé of this research. Finally, chapter seven describes the outlook and limitations of this research.

2 Theoretical part

In the following section, guidance concepts and terms of guidance are defined. Guidance in care and the legal basis are explained. This is followed by a description of the counselling process and the goal of counselling. For an in-depth understanding of communicative competence, the theoretical part includes the approaches of Carl R. Rogers and Paul Watzlawick, as well as an introduction to verbal, non-verbal and paraverbal communication. Furthermore, the counselling competences of the staff of the higher service for health care and nursing are discussed, and nursing counselling in the inpatient oncological setting is dealt with. The importance and role of relatives are also considered in more detail. The structure and process of an oncological counselling session are described in detail.

Cancers are systemic diseases that require holistic, multidisciplinary and long-term treatment of the affected patients. In the WHO European Region, cancer is the second leading cause of death after diseases of the circulatory system. Every year, 2.5 million new cases are diagnosed. Cancer is responsible for about a quarter of the annual deaths (STATISTIK AUSTRIA).

Development of cancer prevalence in Austria since 2002:

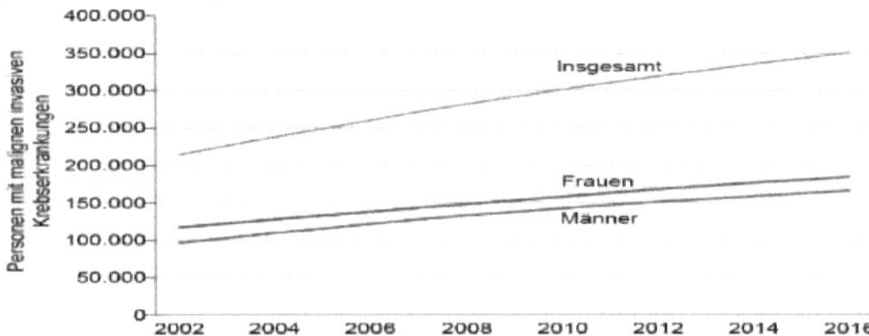

Figure 1: Bundesministerium fur Gesundheit STATISTIK AUSTRIA, Osterreichisches Krebsregister und Todesursachenstatistik (Access: 05.05.2019)

Cancer has an unpredictable course. Corbin & Strauss describe this curve in chronic diseases, which are always associated with an upward and downward or constant direction of movement. The course of a chronic disease is not only determined by the disease itself, but an important role is played by the patients, their relatives and the caregivers themselves. An oncological disease differs in its course dynamics. An alternating sequence of crisis, unstable and stable phases determines the complexity of the demands on the carers during the course of the disease. This in turn enables targeted and comprehensive disease management in medical and nursing care during the course of the disease (cf. Schaeffer/Moers 2008: 6-31).

The diagnosis of cancer triggers feelings of helplessness, anger and despair, but also fear in those affected and their relatives. In addition to the psychological burdens of cancer, patients and their relatives are often faced with financial, professional and social burdens. The nursing care of people with cancer as well as the support of their relatives require high competences on different levels from the staff of the higher service for health care and nursing in oncology. Since oncological patients in particular require a high level of counselling and information, nurses are responsible for providing patients with adequate, comprehensible and up-to-date information about the necessary treatment and care measures (Maiwald/Wecht, 2006: 14).

In oncological care, the importance of information and counselling for patients and their relatives is increasing. The oncological counselling interview in a primary care hospital in Vorarlberg is perceived as a special challenge by the staff of the higher service for health care and nursing. Above all, it involves being able to spontaneously engage in discussions with complex questions with the patients and their relatives. In their professional everyday life, however, the nurses are often overwhelmed in their role as mediator, contact person and confidant, also exhausted, helpless and helpless, but also a lack of self-reflection is recognisable in the exchange with the nurses. Especially after the doctor has given bad news, the nurses are the first contact person for the patients and their relatives. Unconsciously, counselling is carried out by nurses as part of their daily work. This usually takes the form of passing on information and providing guidance in relation to practical care activities. A professional understanding of counselling by nurses is not yet sufficiently developed. Extensive counselling by nurses requires expertise, a certain time frame for implementation and empathic skills in dealing with patients and their relatives. Based on this introduction to the theory of counselling, it can be seen that nurses are required to deal with nursing counselling in the oncological setting in order to develop an in-depth understanding of communication and counselling in nursing.

In order to understand the importance of communication and the relationship between patients, their relatives and caregivers, it is important to look at the principles of care theories. In the following section, three nursing theories are presented which play an important role in nursing counselling:

- **Interaction-oriented theories**

Interactionist theories focus on the attitudes, feelings and actions of patients and carers. Meleis describes characteristics of interaction as validation (Wiedenbach), meeting the patient's needs (Orlando) and being present (Paterson and Zderad) (cf. Schaefer et al, 1997; Meleis, 1999; cited in Koch-Straube, 2008:16f).

The tasks of the nurses thus include the perception and tracing of the illness situation of the patients, empathy and humanity. Personal commitment and participation are further important competences of the nurses in the interactionist nursing theory. The aim is to create an equal relationship between the nurses and the patients, in which the patients have influence and decision-making power.

Needs-based theories

In the needs-based theory, on the other hand, nurses support patients with the aim of regaining autonomy and carrying out the activities of daily living. As a result, self-realisation, self-responsibility and autonomy are considered as outcomes of care, but the personal potential of patients is not taken into account (cf. Abdallah, Henderson; cited in Koch-Straube, 2008: 21f).

- **Outcome-oriented theories**

In the outcome-oriented theory, too, the focus is not on creating a relationship of equal partners. This means that differentiated perspectives, the autonomy and stubbornness of patients are not given any recognition. For a concept of counselling, however, it is necessary that the individuality and subjective views of the patients can be included (cf. Koch-Straube, 2008: 24f).

In the newer concepts of Neumann and Newman, the aim is to understand the illness as a human experience. The role of the nurse is to support this process of awareness. This expansion of consciousness activates the patient to recognise alternatives and to respond in a variety of ways. This is how Newman describes the role of the nurse as a life counsellor. This form of counselling involves more than informing, guiding and giving advice. The concept of counselling in Neumann's and Newman's theories includes psychosocial counselling competences, i.e. activities that do not belong to the nursing-specific competences (cf. Schaeffer et al. 1997: 251; quoted in Koch-Straube, 2008: 27f).

The central basis of caregivers is the encounter with patients, which includes the physical and psychosocial level. This theory of care corresponds to the ideas of the philosophy of holism. A core principle of holism *is "the whole is more than the sum of its parts"*, thus defining the unity of body, mind and spirit in the care of patients.

The oncological counselling interview of the staff of the upper-level service for health care and nursing in a primary care hospital in Vorarlberg includes information about the course of the disease and the management of side effects as well as a psychological, social and pastoral component. This variety of competences shows the complexity of a cancer disease and the resulting individual discussion and counselling that nurses have to do in the oncological setting. Talking, guiding, but also counselling as well as informing, comforting and coaxing receive little attention in nursing. The activity of counselling is taken over by doctors, psychologists, social workers or pastors. Furthermore, the emotional virtues such as patience and empathy, sympathy and warmth are assigned as an essential part of the personality structure of women. They are not professionally acquired knowledge and skills, but are taken for granted and expected of women (cf. Koch-Straube, 1997: 363).

In professional interaction with people, awareness is necessary of why something is said, what technique is used, but also why something is not said. It requires time, practice and reflection on the part of the carer. If done well or poorly, conversational interactions can be remembered by patients and their families as well as by the nurses themselves (cf. Radziewicz & Baile, 2001; Virani, Malloy, Ferrell & Kelly, 2008).

Paul Watzlawick made the statement: "*you cannot not communicate*". This means that every behaviour in an interpersonal situation involves communication. This includes behaviour of all kinds, such as all paralinguistic phenomena, but also body posture and body language, since feelings and emotions are expressed through the body (cf. Watzlawick, 2016: 13f).

Human communication is influenced in terms of content and form by the psychological characteristics of the persons involved. Friedemann Schulz von Thun describes eight different communication styles that correlate with specific personality traits. These include a needy-dependent and helping style. Furthermore, there is a selfless, aggressive-devaluing and proving oneself style. A decisive-controlling and distancing style and a communicative-dramatising style show possible communication disturbances. These communication styles by Friedemann Schulz von Thun result in typical sequences of relationship dynamics, which can lead to a disrupted course of conversation (cf. Elzer/Sciborski, 2007: 156).

In summary, it can be seen that the phenomena of regression and transfer to nurses, triggered by cancer, require a reflective attitude, a balanced nurse-patient relationship and professional communicative competences in leading conversations, so that counselling in the oncological setting can be successful.

2.1 Fundamentals of counselling

In this section, guidance concepts are presented. The term "guidance" as well as guidance in care and the legal basis of guidance are explained in detail. The guidance process and the goal of each guidance are essential points in this section.

Counselling can answer questions and provide guidance, but it can also solve problems and provide security. Making plans and decisions are also part of counselling. Counsellors in all professions have their expert knowledge in their respective counselling fields. Communicating this knowledge in different everyday cultures and to clients is called counselling professionalism. This also includes a basic ability to engage in dialogue with those seeking advice (cf. Schroer, 2010, cited in Rietmann/Sawatzki, 2018: 98).

Nestmann 1997 describes counselling in Germany as the "little sister of therapy". In the USA there are already recognised training and recognition programmes in which counselling is a special discipline of the psychological profession (cf. Nestmann, 1997: 161).

The definitions of counselling must always be related to their scientific reference discipline, which includes psychology, social work and pedagogy. Engel sees the "redefinition of counselling in care" both in the distinction from and in addition to these definitions of counselling (cf. Engel, 2006: 10).

Gorres writes that nurses must be able to acquire and apply communicative, interpretative, strategic and problem-solving competences in addition to action competences (cf. Elzer/Scirboski, 2007: 103).

2.1.1 Counselling concepts

Counselling concepts are characterised according to different emphases in terms of their conception of man, the modification of behaviour and the goals of counselling. The following is an overview of psychological, social science and integrative counselling concepts:

- **Psychological counselling concepts**

Humanistic counselling concepts mean that people are seen in their wholeness, i.e. as an inseparable unity of body, mind and soul. This includes, among others, client-centred talk psychotherapy or non-directive counselling, which was founded by Carl R. Rogers. This approach is discussed in more detail in chapter 2.2.1. The behavioural counselling concepts describe that all behaviour, whether demanding or causing illness, can be learned and thus also unlearned. Sigmund Freud describes the depth psychological approach to counselling, which implies that the unconscious is not directly accessible to the human being. This approach is not designed for counselling in nursing, as it requires therapeutic training. Systemic concepts have developed from family therapy and are characterised by a "solution orientation" in counselling (cf. Koch-Straube, 2008: 104-110).

- **Social science counselling concepts**

Social science counselling concepts are changing from the disease-oriented individualistic view to counselling that includes social and economic life relationships. Concepts of psychosocial counselling developed from this (cf. Sieckendiek et al., 1999: 179; cited in Koch-Straube, 2008: 110f).

- **Integrative counselling**

The basic concepts of integrative counselling are described as co_respondence. This means that the human being is always in relationship with his environment and his fellow human beings. This enables him to develop, survive and understand himself. It is a constantly repeated process of integration (cf. Rahm et al., 1995: 79; quoted in Koch-Straube, 2008:115).

The concepts already mentioned show that in reality a mix of methods is used. This makes it possible to react flexibly to different problem situations. The decisive factor, however, is the knowledge and feeling that a counsellor brings to the table.

2.1.2 Counselling concept

The term "guidance" is a familiar form of communication used in everyday life, which is to be distinguished from professional guidance. The diverse use of the term "counselling" makes a uniform definition difficult. The boundaries between counselling and therapy can be described in such a way that in therapy people with disorders are treated in their personality structure. Counselling, on the other hand, deals with limited problem situations and how to deal with them. Help-oriented everyday speech in professional care should not be confused with counselling, as counselling is carried out in a goal-oriented and methodologically professional manner. Everyday counselling often takes place accidentally in everyday care and is carried out intuitively by the caregivers. In the form of training and information, counselling patient education takes place mainly in the medical and nursing field (cf.

Koch-Straube, 2008: 69).

Counselling is defined as a voluntary, mostly short-term and situational social interaction in non-pathological problem cases between counsellors and those seeking advice, with the aim of developing a decision-making aid for coping with a problem together with the clients in the counselling process (cf. Schwarzer/Posse 1986: 634).

Nestmann defines guidance as professional support that seeks to discover, challenge and sustain social relationships and networks, organisations and institutions, as well as built and natural environments, in a joint process of orientation, planning, decision-making and action. The aim is to enable the development of individuals in formal and informal systems and to achieve a self-determined and self-controlled shaping of everyday life and living. It also involves dealing with the demands and making use of the opportunities for development. However, counselling also involves preventing stresses and crises and tackling them as early as possible so that the consequences for people and systems can be dealt with constructively (cf. Nestmann, 1997: 3334).

Tschudin, on the other hand, distinguishes between professional persons who are employed as counsellors and persons who act as counsellors in their normal activities (cf. Tschudin, 1990: 14).

Koch-Straube describes the concept of guidance as follows:

"The overall aim of counselling is to enable the client to lead a more satisfying and fulfilling life. The term counselling encompasses work with individuals, couples or groups, often but not always referred to as 'clients'. The goals of each counselling relationship vary according to the needs of the client. Counselling is concerned with developmental processes and can address and resolve specific problems, help clients make decisions, manage crises, gain insight and knowledge, work through inner conflicts, improve relationships with others. The counsellor's role is to facilitate the client's work in a way that respects the client's values, personal resources and capacity for self-determination" (BAC, The code of ethics and practice for counsellors, 1993, cited in Koch-Straube 2008: 66).

Engel and Sickendiek point out that counselling is a constantly changing field of activity, which is shaped by social and technical developments in which new problems and challenges can be identified (cf. Engel/Sickendiek 2005: 164).

In summary, counselling can be seen as a form of problem solving, but also as a relationship process between counsellor and counselee. The systemic perspective within the counselling process serves to broaden the perspective and to gain more clarity about one's own problems and their possibilities of coping through the interaction with someone else. It is about identifying existing competences and resources and encouraging them to be used (cf. Koch-Straube, 2007: 228).

2.1.3 Counselling in care

Many successful conversation and counselling situations in care arise from the personal everyday competence of the caregiver and not from a systematic analysis and reflection of care situations and a professionally applied technique. Here, solutions are offered from one's own wealth of experience, and counselling is therefore also defined as lay counselling or everyday counselling, which is characterised by a certain human closeness and a friendly understanding. In relation to care, however, a lack of competence and seriousness can lead to mistrust and a lack of acceptance on the part of patients (Elzer/Sciborski, 2007: 168).

Nurses most often associate counselling with the communication of information and factual content, but in the context of nursing, counselling is also described as a relationship process between nurses, patients and their relatives (cf. Hummel-Gatz/Doll, 2007:n.d.).

Para- or semi-professional counselling in nursing takes place when nurses bring in their expertise in their daily work and pass on this information. Here, the nurse has no counselling training. In contrast, there is professional counselling in nursing, in which an additional training as a counsellor is necessary (cf. Elzer/Sciborski, 2007: 169).

Counselling in nursing differs from social work and social pedagogy in that nurses see illnesses and the associated physical changes and pain as the focus of interaction. Nurses also have an enormous amount of medical knowledge, but little social science knowledge in comparison. The nursing scientist Ulrike Boehnke, for example, speaks of a phenomenological body theory, since the body as an expression of the human self is more than just a body. Boehnke's concept of the body is linked to the concept of the "psychic skin", which includes an interplay between physical contact and the emergence and development of trust. The carer's relation to the body is the reason why care and the emergence of the self - trust, autonomy, initiative and identity - are closely psychodynamically related (cf. Wolfstetter, 1984: 59ff).

Counselling is therefore an integral part of care that contributes to well-being and recovery. Despite all this, counselling is still associated with informing, instructing and training. The limitations of professional counselling in care are insufficient expertise and undeveloped competencies of the nurses and a lack of training. Fear of difficult existential questions can lead to psychological stress. But also a lack of understanding on the part of colleagues and superiors makes counselling in nursing more difficult. Institutional framework conditions also restrict nurses in their counselling activities. In everyday care, there is a lack of time, but also a lack of the right rooms. Multiple-bed rooms make it difficult to establish initial trusting contact with patients. The prerequisite for counselling is, among other things, getting to know each other and openness. This can hardly be achieved during a short stay. The borderline between counselling and therapy is not easy for nurses in complex situations. The danger of being overtaxed and exceeding one's competence should not be disregarded.

2.1.4 Legal basis in counselling

The introduction of the legal basis starts with an overview of the Patient Charter and the rights to education and information of all patients described therein, and a detailed description of the nursing core competences in relation to health counselling and communication in the Federal Law on Health and Nursing Professions in Austria and an extract from the Social Code.

- **Federal Ministry of Labour, Social Affairs, Health and Consumer Protection: Patient Charter and Legal Bases**

The Patient Charter is an agreement between the Federal Government and the Länder pursuant to Art. 15a B-VG. The Patient Charter describes the basic rights of patients. Patient dignity, self-determination, information and support of patients are the four most important foundations of the Patient Charter. The right to self-determination and information means that patients must be informed in advance about types of diagnosis and treatment as well as their risks and consequences. Furthermore, the right to be informed about the state of health, but also about the necessary cooperation in the treatment and therapy-supportive lifestyle. Treatment only takes place with the consent of the patient or a representative or in case of imminent danger (Article 17). Patients decide what is to happen. In the event of inability to act, it is possible to draw up a patient's declaration of consent (Patient's Charter, accessed: 23.05.2019).

- **The Health Care and Nursing Act**

The **nursing core competences in § 14** (1) and (2) include the autonomous activity of nursing in all forms of care and care levels of prevention, health demand and health counselling within the framework of nursing, as well as the organisation and implementation of training. Furthermore, the nursing core competences include theory- and concept-guided interviewing and communication (GukG, version of 25.05.2019).

The **multiprofessional area of competence in § 16** (3) of the higher service for health care and nursing includes nursing expertise in health counselling, interprofessional networking, information transfer and knowledge management, as well as the coordination of the treatment and care process, including ensuring the continuity of treatment.

§ Section 17 (1) contains **setting- and target group-specific specialisations** in which hospice and palliative care is listed (GukG, version of 25.05.2019).

Hospice and palliative care in § 22b describes the care and support of people with a progressive, incurable and therefore life-threatening illness, as well as the care of their relatives, with the background of achieving an understanding of illness while preserving self-determination and the patient's will to achieve an improved quality of life. Furthermore, palliative care includes counselling and/or training of the patients and their relatives in dealing with the symptoms and forward planning to record the wishes and needs for the last phase of life. Close cooperation and communication with different disciplines is therefore a prerequisite in the care of palliative patients.

- The Social Code (SGB XI), Book Eleven, Social Long-Term Care Insurance

§ 7a SGB XI Care counselling includes the following:

"(1) Persons, ... are entitled to individual counselling and assistance by a care advisor in the selection and use of social benefits provided for by federal or Land law as well as other offers of help which are aimed at supporting people with care, provision or support needs (care counselling); a competent care advisor or other counselling centre should be named immediately by the long-term care insurance funds before the first counselling session. The guidelines according to §17 paragraph 1a are authoritative for the procedure, the implementation and the contents of the long-term care counselling" (SGB XI, accessed on 28.05.2019).

The legal anchoring of counselling shows that counselling in care goes far beyond its field.

2.1.5 Guidance as a process

The guidance process is often dynamic, because the individual phases overlap, but also merge or repeat. There are different phase models in the literature, which differ in the number of phases and their content (cf. Engel 2006: 49; Mutzeck 2008: 21; Gittler-Hebestreit 2006: 39).

The WHO describes the care process in counselling as a relationship between patients and carers with an active involvement in the planning and implementation of their own nursing care (cf.
World Health Organisation, 1980: n.d.)

The four stages of the guidance process in integrative guidance consist of the initial phase or naming, the action phase or experiencing, the integration phase or reflecting and the reorientation phase, testing (cf. Koch-Straube, 2008: 122).

Engel, however, describes the counselling process as a goal-oriented method of analysing, planning, implementing and reviewing, which is carried out together with the patient in the form of a dialogue, similar to the nursing process (cf. Engel, 2006: 49).

An advisory process can therefore be compared to the care process, in which the following steps are necessary to carry out measures. The first step is to analyse the current situation and to clarify the initial situation. The second step is the planning of interventions, taking into account the resources of the patients and their relatives. The third step is the final evaluation. Nurses often do not perceive the activity of counselling as a continuous task. As a result, counselling measures are not documented and thus not regarded as professional nursing activities (cf. Huper/Hellige, 2007: 102).

The tasks and responsibilities of nursing in the context of holistic rehabilitative process care in Krohwinkel's (2007) management model include teaching, counselling and guiding as an integral part. In her model, the patient and his/her relatives are placed at the centre of what happens (cf. Krohwinkel, 2007: 38).

Interaction and communication are a central part of counselling. In expert counselling, specialised nurses provide their knowledge and experience. This expert counselling takes place, among other things, in the oncological setting between the patients, their relatives and the nurse within the framework of an oncological counselling session. In this process counselling, the nurse sees him/herself as a supporter and supporter of a pending development during the disease process. Oncological patients and their relatives need time and space for discussion,

which serve as information and guidance, but also as motivation during the disease process. Coping with the disease also requires supportive or so-called **coping language** when dealing with oncology patients and their relatives. For nurses in the oncology setting, the counselling process consists of informing, such as explaining a therapy plan, but also defining and explaining interventions of side effects during and after chemotherapy are parts of an **informative conversation**. **Guiding talks** can be relaxation techniques for the patients, but also their relatives, during the therapy. **Motivational talks** by the nurses can be supportive and helpful and are an important part for the patients during and after the therapy.

In summary, it can be seen that counselling is a component of the care process. In 2007 Hellige/Huper described counselling in parallel to the care process. They describe that guidance is a process-oriented measure in the care process, but also vice versa.

2.1.6 Aim of the counselling

Counselling is a legal requirement for staff in the upper echelons of health care and nursing, as described in more detail in chapter 2.1.4.

Frose describes the requirements of counselling as complex, as it requires communication skills such as active listening and empathic action as well as up-to-date expert knowledge on the part of the counsellor. The goals of counselling are individually adapted to the person concerned and must be clearly defined (cf. Frose, 2010: 36).

It is crucial that the action competence of those seeking advice is demanded in the counselling so that a solution to a specific problem situation can be given through the method of imparting knowledge (cf. Schaeffer, 2008: 6-8f).

Aron Antonovsky understands health as a process of confrontation between factors that protect or burden health. Antonovsky describes the goal of counselling in care as an increase in coherence. A feeling of coherence is a term from salutogenesis, it is about the question of what keeps people healthy. The feeling of coherence means (cf. Koch-Straube, 2008: 216):

• Understandability - understanding the demands of life, which means that they can be explained and interpreted.

• Manageability - the ability to cope through one's own personal competence and problem-solving skills.

• Meaningfulness - changes are seen as a challenge, are perceived as meaningful

An increase in coherence leads to better compliance and coping of the patient, but also self-activity and health are improved. The goal is thus not to solve the problem but to help the individual to develop so that he/she can cope with the present problem and the later consequences in a better integrated way (cf. Rogers, 1999: 36).

2.2 Basics of communicative competences

This section provides an insight into client-centred communication according to Carl R. Rogers and human communication according to Karl Watzlawick as well as an introduction to verbal, non-verbal and para-verbal communication.

In the care of oncological patients during their stay in hospital, there are many situations in which patients, relatives and nurses have to talk to each other. The organisation of helping and counselling conversations is an important part of everyday care. Carers are therefore important contact persons in a constructive communication process. The different forms of conversations show that communicative competences and counselling skills are necessary to cope with social tasks. Numerous concepts of conversation and counselling in nursing refer to the approach of Carl R. Rogers. In order to conduct consultations and conversations with oncological patients and their relatives, nurses should analyse communication styles in order to establish a connection to oncological care (cf. Thomann 2004: 344).

In the following, the client-centred approach to counselling and psychotherapy according to Carl Rogers, and Karl Watzlawick's human communication are introduced.

2.2.1 Client-centred conversation according to Carl R. Rogers

Carl R. Rogers (1902-1987) was born in Illinois, USA. He studied agriculture, theology and psychology. In the 1940s he developed non-directive counselling, which was later defined as client-centred therapy. Non-directive counselling states that therapists let the client take the initiative in the course of the conversation. In client-centred therapy, the therapist is oriented towards the client's world of experience. In the 1950s and 1960s, the theory of Carl Rogers was made known and further developed in Europe by Reinhard Tausch. The theoretical approach of Carl R. Rogers is based on a humanistic view of man. This implies that the human being is regarded as a holistic being whose goal is self-realisation. Rogers assumed that every person is capable of using his or her abilities to the best of his or her ability so that all his or her needs can be satisfied (cf. Rogers, 1976: n.d.).

The basic hypothesis according to Rogers is that people have the ability to understand themselves and the way they act, and thus to change. In the case of psychological and physical impairments, his abilities are developed in a therapeutic relationship. A non-judgemental attitude towards the client is therefore necessary so that counsellors can turn to them emotionally. The focus is on the process of the relationship. Clients act on their own responsibility.

Client-centred theory is a theory of the process by which change is brought about in persons and their behaviour (cf. Rogers, 1961a: n.d.).

Roger's approach is a phenomenological one, which is concerned with the description and appearance of clients and not with analysis (cf. Elzer/Sciborski, 2007: 87).

These assumptions are explained as follows:

1   Autonomy and interdependence (social interdependence)

In his development, man strives for independence and takes responsibility for his own life. This self-responsibility leads to the fact that man can also take responsibility for the community. Only the discovery of personal responsibility and that one can change oneself will contribute to necessary changes in the environment (cf. Rogers 1940, Groddeck 2002: 79, quoted in Elzer /Sciborski 2007: 83).

2   The self-realisation

Self-realisation and the need for growth are assumed to be the driving forces of the organism, which allow existing abilities to further develop and differentiate (cf. Rogers, 1940, Groddeck 2002: 79, quoted in Elzer /Sciborski 2007: 83).

3   The goal and the sense orientation

Humanistic values such as freedom, justice, dignity and security of existence shape a person's life. An awareness between an inner and an outer reality is purposeful (cf. Rogers 1940, Groddeck 2002: 79, quoted in Elzer /Sciborski 2007: 83).

4   The wholeness

Holism implies that counselling does not intervene in the client's life, but is supportive and helpful. This leads to clients feeling safe, free of fear and empowered (cf. Rogers 1940, Groddeck 2002: 79, quoted in Elzer /Sciborski 2007: 83).

In summary, this means that the client-centred approach's view of human beings includes autonomy and interdependence. Carl R. Rogers understands this to mean that people develop an active self in order to take responsibility for their own lives and thus also for the community. He describes the self-realisation or self-actualisation tendency as the basic driving force of the organism, which can be further developed and balanced in constant exchange with the social environment. Rogers also describes humanistic values such as freedom, justice and human dignity as the goal and orientation of meaning. Finally, he cites the wholeness of feeling and reason, of body and soul (cf. Rogers/Schmid, 1991: 214ff).

In counselling, the focus is not only on nursing expertise, but on understanding and appreciating the patients and their relatives in the respective situation, so that a professional relationship can be established. Rogers describes the basic attitude in counselling as follows:

The Basic Approach of Person-Centred Conversation Leadership

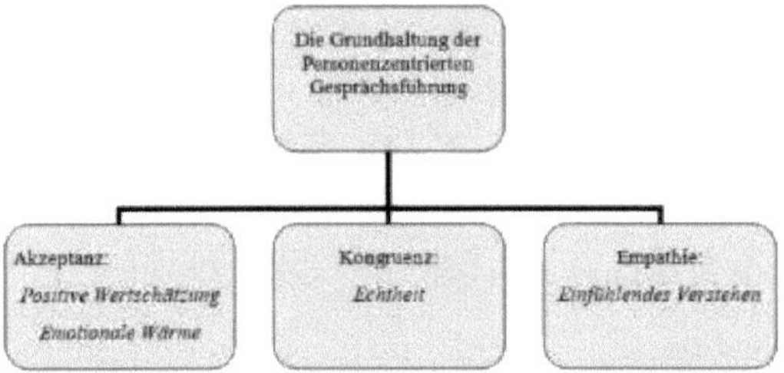

Figure 2: The basic attitude of Person-Centred Conversation Leadership (own illustration)

The three basic variables of the client-centred concept according to Carl R. Rogers include positive regard, authenticity and unconditional acceptance. This means that clients are recognised as persons with their own values and respected in their individuality. The inner thinking and feeling of the counsellor are the prerequisites for an empathic and appreciative congruence between the counsellor and the client. Another basic variable is empathetic understanding, in which the counsellors put themselves in the client's emotional world (cf. Elzer/Sciborski, 2007: 84f).

The basic attitude of counselling is characterised by empathic, non-possessive warmth, sympathy and acceptance. The importance of communication and empathy in the therapy process has been scientifically studied. It was shown that treated persons judged a therapy more strongly according to the communication competence of the therapists and whether they responded to their needs (cf. Dehn-Hindenberg, 2007: 26-33).

In summary, this means that in counselling a human contact can be established between the counsellor and the client in which the client feels safe and accepted and feelings can be freely expressed. The result is that the client recognises and accepts him/herself in the experience of his/her own feelings. The counsellor's task is to guide the client and give supportive information so that the client can continue on his/her own. These basic attitudes exclude certain negative communicative behaviours, which Kris Cole (2003: 158-166) has called "*The Ten Deadly Wounds of Communication*". These include judging, moralising or making ironic remarks (cf. Elzer/Sciborski, 2007: 81ff).

This participatory and supportive attitude makes the client-centred approach suitable for conducting conversations and counselling in care. This approach is therefore of great importance in the oncological setting. The humanistic counselling approaches, which include the concept of non-directive counselling according to Rogers, originated in humanistic psychology. Rogers' theory of personhood causes self-healing and self-actualising powers to be released between a counsellor and a client. In relation to a conversation in an oncological setting, it is therefore particularly important that nurses create a climate of respect, authenticity and understanding so that these self-actualisation forces are activated and positively support the course of the disease of oncological patients and their relatives. Rogers describes the verbalisation of emotional experience contents as particularly important. He verbalises what he has understood and felt from clients. This formulation of the content of experiences is also evident in dealing with oncological patients and their relatives. Therefore, nurses should refrain from any kind of influencing and steering of patients in conversations or counselling, so that more autonomy instead of dependency and self-esteem can be released.

In client-centred counselling, Rogers defines **active listening** and **paraphrasing** as a technical form of intervention in leading the conversation. The repetition of the most important thoughts and feelings by the counsellor is defined as paraphrasing or mirroring the counsellor's own performances. Body language signals interested and attentive listening. Verbal interruptions can influence the client's train of thought. The counsellor's addressing of non-verbal behaviour as well as asking questions in case of ambiguity complete the conversation. The counsellor approaches the situation with open questions (who? how? what?). Silence and pauses are also important elements of a counselling session. However, the non-directive attitude of the counsellor is crucial, which aims to allow patients to develop their own authentic activities (cf.

Elzer/Sciborski, 2007: 86-87).

2.2.2 Human communication according to Paul Watzlawick

Paul Watzlawick (1921-2007) was born in Austria. He was a communication scientist, psychotherapist, psychoanalyst, sociologist, philosopher and author. His communication theory is based on the five axioms, which state that communication always has an effect on the behaviour of clients and counsellors.

1   Axiom on the impossibility of not communicating

Watzlawick assumes that one cannot not communicate. Every behaviour in an interpersonal situation involves communication. This means that even through silence or non-communication, communication takes place. As soon as people perceive each other, communication takes place intentionally or unintentionally. This includes behaviour of all kinds, such as all paralinguistic phenomena (tone of voice, laughter, sighing), but also body posture and body language, since feelings and emotions are expressed through the body (cf. Watzlawick, 2016: 13).

2   Axiom on the content and relationship aspect of communication

Communication is divided into a content aspect (WHAT) and a relationship aspect (HOW). The predominantly verbal content aspect comprises factual information, in contrast to the verbal and non-verbal relationship aspect, which specifies how this information is to be understood by the receiver and how the sender defines the relationship between him/herself and the receiver. This means that if the interlocutors have a stable relationship, different opinions can be allowed without the relationship suffering or breaking down. The prerequisite is positive and appreciative interaction (cf. Watzlawick, 2016: 16).

3   Axiom for the punctuation of event sequences

Communication is a circular exchange without a clear beginning or end. Cause and effect lie in the interpretation of the communication partners. Watzlawick assumes that we have our own reality and hold it to be true, and that this subjective reality determines our actions. This can lead to different understandings or misunderstandings in the communication relationship (cf. Watzlawick, 2016: 20).

4   Axiom on digital vs. analogue communication

Watzlawick divides communication into speaking to each other, the digital statement and the analogue statement of body language, gestures and facial expressions, body posture and context. Misunderstandings can arise when patients are no longer able to communicate digitally, as sign language or gestures can lead to misinterpretations (cf. Watzlawick, 2016: 24f).

5   Axiom on symmetrical vs. complementary communication

The two types of relationships represent relationships based on either equality or difference. Symmetrical relationships are characterised by the pursuit of equality and the reduction of differences between the partners. Complementary interactions, on the other hand, are based on mutually complementary differences. Both forms can stabilise in a good relationship and even alternate or complement each other. When dealing with seriously ill patients, it is therefore important that the relationship between nurses and patients is not one-sided, but that activating and patient-oriented care is practised (cf. Watzlawick, 2016: 32ff).

Watzlawick's statements imply that failures in communication are the rule. The difficulties in communication are that each person relies on his or her personal perception and believes it to be true and real. This means that communication can be complicated by misunderstandings and misinterpretations. In his opinion, communication can be successful if the communication partners go beyond themselves, so that communication is possible on a further meta-level. With his theory, Watzlawick wanted to show that it is impossible "not to communicate" (cf. Elzer/Sciborski, 2007: 115-117).

In summary, Rogers' rules of communication refer to empathy. He describes that it is important to empathise with the person you are talking to and to communicate what you have understood back to the other person. This model according to Rogers contains the basic question: How can people understand each other better in the process of communication? It is a model of the perspective of the interlocutor. In contrast, Watzlawick asks the question on the basis of his five axioms: How can a common reality be formed in communication? In this communication model, the perception of reality is in the foreground (cf. Rohner/Schurz, 2012: 32).

2.2.3 Verbal, non-verbal and paraverbal communication

Communication takes place at different levels of communication. Verbal communication is the actual language, while body language and localisation are called non-verbal communication. The involvement of all the senses, such as sight, hearing, touch and smell, are among the characteristics of non-verbal communication. Possibilities of non-verbal expression include facial expressions, gestures, posture, touching, distance, laughing, but also silence or status symbols such as clothing and hairstyle. The loudness of the voice, the pitch, the tone of voice and the speed of speech are all part of the paraverbal form of expression in communication. These characteristics shape the content of information through the way something is said (cf. Ekert/Ekert, 2010: 203).

In oncology nursing, talking and listening are important components of non-verbal communication that contribute to a successful relationship between the nurses and patients and their relatives. The way a carer speaks also facilitates a trusting relationship. Whether too soft or too loud, both can lead to a lack of trust in the carer (cf. Kreddig & Zohra 2013: 202).

2.3 Counselling competence in care

This section deals with the definition of the term "competence" and a detailed description of the professional competence of nursing which enables successful counselling in nursing.

The term competence is derived from the Latin verb *competere* (to come together) and the noun *competentia* (aptitude), and means the coming together of different abilities to form a competence to act. The ability to express oneself and how language can be used in social situations is defined in linguistics as linguistic competence and performance (cf. Chomsky 1969; Duden 2001a, cited in Elzer/Sciborski, 2007: 41f).

In order to be able to offer counselling, nurses need to expand their competences. In counselling, the focus is not only on nursing expertise, but also on understanding and appreciating the patients and their relatives in the respective situation, so that a professional relationship can be established. According to Koch-Straube, the prerequisites for successful counselling in nursing are knowledge of the theoretical foundations of counselling and methodological competence, so that the counselling process can be designed in a goal-oriented and systematic way. But also the ability to perceive the patients and their relatives individually and the willingness to develop and use oneself for understanding situations is a component of the competences of nurses in counselling. Crucial, however, is the ability to share knowledge and information, but also instructions and experiences, in a more appropriate way with those involved (cf. Koch-Straube, 2008:182).

The professional action competences are divided into four basic competences, the interface of which is communicative competence (Elzer/Sciborski, 2007: 45f):

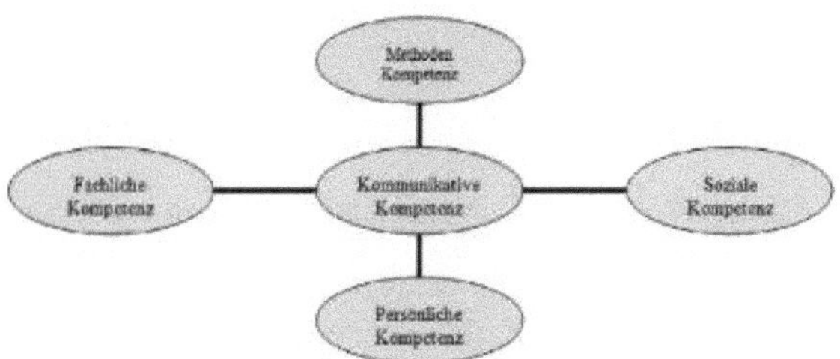

Figure 3: The professional competences in nursing (own representation)

2.3.1 Professional competence

Professional competence with regard to nursing is acquired through nursing training, further training, studies and several years of professional practice. Professional competences include the special knowledge about the operative knowledge of a profession (cf. Olk, 1989: 89).

2.3.2 Methodological competence

Methodological competence in relation to nursing includes specific nursing methods and techniques, including their implementation.

2.3.3 Social competence

Social competence in nursing involves nurses being aware of their professional role and carrying out and being rewarded for their work in a professional manner.

2.3.4 Personal competence

In relation to nursing, personal competence describes motivation in the profession as well as empathic skills in dealing with patients. But it also includes the nurses' own ability to reflect.

The interface of the four basic competences is called communicative competence. As the core of communicative competence, Jurgen Habermas (1971, 1976, 1981) mentions *"the claim to reasonableness"*, *"the claim to truth"*, as well as *"the claim to truthfulness"* and *"the claim to correctness"* (cf. Elzer/Sciborski, 2007: 47-48).

Counselling in care can only succeed if the competences are sufficiently developed so that a need for counselling can be recognised in time and the counselling process can be managed. Demanding these competences through targeted education, training and further education as well as a reflected professional practice is necessary so that nurses can fulfil their counselling function. The necessary working conditions for shaping a counselling process must also be supported. The following section therefore presents a detailed description of nursing counselling in the oncological setting.

2.4 Nursing counselling in the inpatient "oncological setting

This section defines and describes the inpatient oncology setting as well as the contents of a nursing oncology consultation in a primary care hospital in Vorarlberg.

When we talk about oncology, we are really talking about the study of tumour diseases, cancers. Oncological patients have to attend many therapy and control appointments during their treatment. All these journeys are arduous for a sick person. The oncological treatment of those affected should take place as close as possible to their place of residence to make it easier for them. In the described primary care hospital in Vorarlberg, the patients are accompanied from the initial consultation to the initiation of the diagnostic steps to the preparation of a treatment plan (as well as the resulting therapy phases). Additional tasks include aftercare and the entire drug therapy including chemotherapy, immunotherapy and targeted tumour therapy, which includes radiation and surgery. The patients are treated and accompanied in all phases of their illnesses. This basic care in the treatment of tumour diseases and the support in the palliative situation enable targeted and comprehensive care of the patients in the oncological setting of the described primary care hospital in Vorarlberg.

The term "setting" comes from English and means environment, framework. The original term comes from analytical psychotherapy. The setting is characterised by the purpose of the situation. Furthermore, framework conditions and the agreement between the participants are the prerequisite for a helping relationship to develop. The setting influences the quality and the limits of a conversation (cf. Elzer/Sciborski, 2007: 123).

Based on the treatment process of cancer in an oncological setting, the different counselling situations for nurses are defined in more detail in the following paragraph.

2.4.1 Cancer treatment process

Communication begins with the suspicion of a cancer diagnosis and continues through all phases of treatment, follow-up care and the end-of-life phase. Oncological counselling by nurses will be discussed in more detail on the basis of the individual phases of a cancer disease, so that an understanding can be built up of which competences nurses must have in order to provide patient-centred care.

Furthermore, the role of relatives will be discussed, as they also need professional support and counselling in all phases of the disease.

Phase 1: Learning about the diagnosis

In the described primary care hospital in Vorarlberg, oncological patients are informed about their tumour disease and the current therapy plan within the framework of a medical consultation. The doctor and the patient as well as the relatives are present at this medical consultation. Ideally, a nurse is also present. When delivering a diagnosis, honesty and trust between the doctor and the patient are essential to reduce fear. False hopes should be avoided in this discussion so that those affected can make their decision realistically for the future (cf. Langkafel/Ludke, 2008: 42f).

The oncology nurse also plays an important role as a mediator between doctors and patients. In an understandable language, ambiguities can be communicated to the patients and their relatives. Oncology nurses are often the first point of contact for patients after they have been diagnosed with cancer. A close relationship develops between the nurses and patients, but also with their relatives. These reactions of *not wanting to admit, only understanding in part* or not *hearing or forgetting most things* lead to misunderstandings in the communication between those affected, the doctors and nurses (cf. Weyland, 2013: 51).

Phase 2: The treatment

After the diagnosis of cancer, the patients enter the phase of processing, which means an extraordinary and completely new situation in their lives. The individual medical stages in the treatment and every change in the state of health result in numerous questions for the patients and their relatives in coping with the disease. Dealing with cancer is made easier when there is openness between relatives about the situation at hand.

According to the study results of the S3 guidelines, Psychooncology in Adult Cancer Patients, the need for information hardly changes during the course of treatment. Those affected most often name a need for support in dealing with fears about the progression of the disease and a changed body image. Depression, but also hope and meaning in coping with the disease, and worries about the family and its future are aspects that are mentioned. Control over one's own life and a good quality of life are further goals. Fear of pain and dealing with exhaustion, questions about dying as well as problems in everyday life and working life require special information support.

These complex issues require special language skills on the part of oncology nurses. People with cancer and their relatives need to be able to talk about their fears (cf. Oncology guideline programme, accessed: 05.05.2019).

Not only are psycho-oncological counselling skills required of oncology nurses, but also intervention recommendations for the most important symptoms of cancer require appropriate expertise. The management of side effects and their supportive measures during and after chemotherapy are aspects of the oncology nurses' consultation. The most common side effects, such as nausea and vomiting, as well as fatigue and exhaustion, loss of appetite and inflammation of the oral mucosa, can be alleviated or reversed during therapy with supportive measures.

Also, many patients and their relatives are already pre-informed via the internet. This is one of the new challenges for the oncology nurse, as patients and their relatives already bring a lot of information from the internet into a counselling session.

Phase 3: The recovery phase

After completion of the treatment, the patients are examined at regular intervals in the sense of a special aftercare programme. These check-ups serve to ensure that side effects of the treatment, but also a recurrence of the disease, can be detected in time to intervene. These check-ups cause great anxiety for those affected. In the oncological setting, patients are already very anxious days before their check-up appointments, as they expect bad findings at any time. These fears of progression are common among patients and their relatives, and are therefore a particular challenge for nurses in the oncology setting. Their task is, among other things, to talk to and support those affected.

Studies from Australia and Sweden show that the use of oncology nurses in follow-up care is equivalent to that of doctors in terms of safety and complications for various tumour diseases. However, patients are more satisfied when oncology nurses carry out the follow-up checks (cf. Zukunft der Onkologiepflege, 2018: 182).

Phase 4: The occurrence of a relapse

If a cancer disease is advanced, stabilisation of the course of the disease is a primary goal. This means that together with the patients and their relatives, an improved quality of life is achieved through targeted pain and symptom management. In this phase, the counselling of the nurses includes not only interventions to reduce the side effects of chemotherapy, but also the alleviation of psychological, social and spiritual problems. Unlike at the time of initial diagnosis, those affected have a wealth of knowledge and an idea of what the new treatment will be like. Fear, anger and uncertainty dominate and can lead to patients becoming suspicious and sceptical of caregivers (cf. Hausmann 2014: 131f).

Phase 5: The terminal-palliative phase

This last stage of life includes the care of palliative patients and the care of the dying, an important part of the discussions in the oncological setting between the patients, their relatives and the nurses. Accompanying and caring for patients and their relatives in the last days or hours requires a special sensitivity on the part of the carers. For many relatives it is important to accompany or be close to the patient until his/her death. In order for the relatives to be able to provide appropriate support, preventive explanations adapted to the situation and competent counselling by the caregivers are required.

2.4.2 The role of relatives in the oncology setting

The diagnosis of cancer also triggers a shock for relatives. Carers in the oncological setting often see them only in their function as carers and discussion partners of the patients. What is overlooked is that relatives are also affected in the sense that they are threatened with the loss of an important person. Therefore, it makes sense to also be available to relatives as a discussion partner. The tasks of oncology nurses in coping with the disease are not only to accompany the patients, but also to actively involve their relatives in the disease process.

During the medical consultation and the preparation of the treatment plan, it is helpful if relatives can be present, with the consent of the person concerned.

At the same time, relatives are burdened themselves. They need support above all through discussion and respectful handling of their situation. Relatives contribute to enabling patient-centred care in the oncological setting. They accompany the patients to their examinations or during chemotherapy, which makes them a great support for the patients, but also for carers in the oncology setting (cf. Die Osterreichische Krebshilfe, 2018: 24).

2.4.3 Structure and course of a counselling interview in the inpatient "oncological setting

In principle, counselling is process-oriented. This means, among other things, that nurses in the oncological setting are able to directly address difficulties that are common among oncologists (cf. Baumer, 2008: 343).

Every professional conversation in the oncological setting requires a planning of external and internal factors for the communication process. In the described primary care hospital in Vorarlberg, the following prerequisites are necessary for a professional counselling conversation between the nurses and the patients and their relatives:

- **Premises**

It is an advantage for the interview if there is a specially equipped interview or single room on the ward. If this is not possible and the interview takes place in a shared room, fellow patients and visitors should be asked to leave the room for the duration of the interview. This is not only necessary for reasons of data protection, but also so that the persons concerned can feel safe and undisturbed. The radio, television and telephone are switched off to create a quiet and relaxed atmosphere for the conversation. A sign on the door saying "*Please do not enter*" can also be helpful.

The colleagues are informed so that the carer can talk in peace (cf. Elzer/Sciborski, 2007: 195f).

- **Preparation of an oncological counselling interview**

The preparation of an oncology consultation depends on whether the nurse has already been able to be present at the medical consultation. This is helpful because the nurse has already received some important information about the planned therapy, such as whether it is an adjuvant or palliative treatment of the cancer. They also already know the patient and relatives, which can be a confidence booster when starting a conversation. Preparation includes the therapy plan, the management of side effects of chemotherapy and the most important organisational procedures. It also makes sense for the nurse to plan an appointment with the patients and their relatives in advance, so that they can also prepare themselves. This is important because many questions arise after the initial diagnosis and the patients and their families are uncertain. This gives them the opportunity to write down questions in advance and bring them to the planned discussion (cf. Hausmann, 2014: 208).

- **Start of an oncological counselling session**

When starting a counselling session, it is important to have an upright sitting position and eye contact with the people concerned. A round table or sitting diagonally across from each other is most comfortable for all involved during counselling. If the patient is lying down, the counsellor and relatives should be positioned at the side of the bed with a chair so that all partners are at the same eye level. The content and duration of the counselling session is determined at the beginning, after the counsellor has introduced him/herself by name. With a simple question to the patient, the nurse can open the conversation, such as: *"What do you know about your doctor's consultation and what is unclear to you?* From this feedback, an experienced nurse can see where to start in order to make professional counselling a success. Listening and paraphrasing at the beginning of the discussion relaxes the situation between the discussion partners and helps the counsellor to approach the person concerned in an empathetic and appreciative way (cf. Hausmann, 2014: 208).

- **Contents of an oncological counselling session**

Oncological counselling by nurses includes the course of treatment as well as side effects of therapy and disease, such as nausea, vomiting, tiredness and fatigue, but also loss of appetite and inflammation of the oral mucosa. Late effects of the therapy can be hair loss and polyneuropathies. Furthermore, preventive measures are discussed with the patients during the therapy, but also how everyday life can be managed. Support in dealing with their family members, especially children, is also part of nursing counselling. The mediation with the different network partners is also part of it, for example the cancer support, psycho-oncological support, regional social services and self-help groups in the country. Organisational content can include the next appointments, planned examinations, but also additional visits to the family doctor. In this phase, the involvement of relatives is often very helpful, as they can accompany the patient during examinations or therapy and thus support him/her. But also information and the correct handling of complementary measures are available in the care counselling. Unclear terms and long sentences should be avoided. Points that are important in the conversation should be repeated again (cf. Hausmann 2014, p. 208).

It is also not always possible to cover all the content in the first counselling session. Information about issues can be conveyed in different ways and supplemented with brochures and leaflets so that patients and their relatives have the opportunity to deal with the information more intensively even after a counselling session. However, it is crucial to allow enough time for questions, but also for emotional discussions during the counselling session.

- **Ending an oncology counselling session**

The end of the conversation is similar to the beginning, again with a question to the person concerned: *"I can imagine that this situation is not easy for you. Is there anything else that would be important to you in today's conversation?"* Repeating the most important cornerstones of the counselling content is also a step towards ending a conversation. If the time was too short, another appointment should be arranged. A respectful and appreciative conclusion is a prerequisite for the person concerned, but also for the carers in the counselling (cf. Hausmann, 2014: 208).

For a better understanding of this research, the researcher has described in detail the nursing consultation in the oncology setting. This serves to provide an understanding of the choice of methods for this research process in the empirical part of this thesis.

3 Empirical part

This chapter begins with an introduction to qualitative research. This is followed by a detailed description of the methodological procedure. Each of the sub-chapters begins with a theoretical treatment of the respective methods, and is then devoted to their practical implementation, whereby theory and practice overlap in places for the sake of clarity.

3.1 Qualitative research

Qualitative research has its roots in philosophy and is based on the ideas that pay to the humanities. The latter grasp their object as a whole and interpret it instead of measuring it. It can be deduced from this that for qualitative research reality does not only consist of objectively measurable facts. Reality is understood to be research approaches that deal with people and the reality they experience. The meaning and the connections that are created in the course of social interaction are in the foreground. The subjective perception of reality and truth cannot be measured objectively, but only through subjective understanding (cf. Mayer, 2014: 73).

In qualitative research, the phenomena to be researched are not broken down into individual parts and/or taken out of context. The holistic and subjective approach makes it possible to experience and understand human experience. With the help of semi-standardised or non-standardised instruments, an open data collection is carried out. Data evaluation is an interpretative method of descriptions. The aim of qualitative research is therefore to form theories and concepts (cf. Mayer, 2014: 74).

Due to the research question, the researcher of this thesis decided to use a qualitative research approach in order to gain an insight into topics in the context of a nursing counselling session of the staff of the higher service for health care and nursing in the oncological setting. The experiences of the nurses in counselling situations with patients and their relatives are subjective experiences from which insights are gained. The perspective of the nurses, their reality and their experience during a counselling session with patients and their relatives in the oncology setting are the focus of this research. Six interviews with nurses in the oncology setting are conducted and recorded with a dictation machine and IPAD. The verbatim, but smoothed (i.e. High German) transcription will be analysed and evaluated with the help of Grounded Theory (see chapter 3.2). The study was conducted in the direct research field of an oncology department in a primary care hospital in Vorarlberg. An open approach and a narrative interview guide for data collection describe the inductive and theory-developing procedure of this research work. The aim of this research is to experience, identify and understand basic issues that come up in the context of a nursing counselling session in an oncology setting, as well as the focus on difficulties, obstacles and the unexpected in the context of a counselling session.

In order to develop an object-related theory in this research, grounded theory is used in the context of qualitative research, which is described in more detail in the next section.

3.2 Introduction to Grounded Theory

The research style of grounded theory can be classified as social science hermeneutics. This deals with scientific and everyday understanding and interpretation. The term hermeneutics is derived from the Greek "hermeneuein" and means to state, interpret, overlook. The comprehension of human behavioural patterns refers to hermeneutic understanding. The process of understanding is examined and structured. It is not based on a uniform and universally accepted theory. The basic idea of this process of interpretation describes the hermeneutic circle. This implies that one can only understand a text if a certain pre-understanding is already present. The understanding gained from the text thus has an effect on the previous understanding, which is constantly expanded. This results in a spiral movement of knowledge through a repeated circular movement between a priori assumptions (pre-understanding) and the phenomena in the field of research. The hermeneutic circle thus means that the understanding of parts results from the whole, and the understanding of the whole results from the parts (cf. Lamnek/Krell, 2016: 71ff).

For the researcher of this study, this means that with each reading process, the understanding of the text as a whole and in its individual statements improves. An essential characteristic of the creative development of knowledge is the switching back and forth between "two worlds", namely practical action and reflection (cf. Breuer, 2010: 46ff).

Strauss describes the spiral research process as iterative-cyclical, which serves the development of knowledge. A continuous back and forth between data collection, coding and theory building alternates in different sequences. Jumps, such as a renewed attention to already coded material with a different focus background, make sense (cf. Breuer et al, 2009: 55).

Strauss and Glaser refer to the evaluation or text interpretation process as coding, which means breaking down and conceptualising the generated data. All occurrences that seem relevant are named, explained and discussed in the data. In order to ultimately develop a theory from the raw data, the researcher can make use of three types of coding - open, axial and selective coding (see chapter 3.5.3). At the end of the coding process, the researcher receives a list of concepts (cf. Bohm, 1994: 126f).

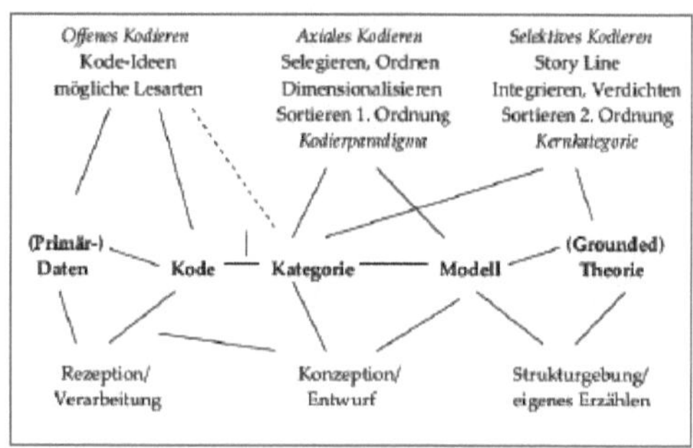

Figure 4: Coding process in systematic order (cf. Breuer et al., 2009: 76)

The figure above shows that the coding process is to be understood as a constant back and forth, forward and backward between data collection, the formation of concepts and model testing as well as a final reflection (cf. Breuer et al, 2009: 69).

Glaser and Strauss point out that data should be collected and analysed simultaneously. This means that already after the first interview with the respondent, and the first field observations by the researcher, this investigation of the analysis process has begun. This means that the following interpretations and observations are carried out on the basis of analytical questions and hypotheses about categories and their relationships (Glaser/Strauss, 1998: 52ff).

The core process of grounded theory involves theory development through concept formation, which takes place on the basis of data analysis (coding) according to a concept-indicator model. The visible everyday phenomena are seen as indicators of underlying, invisible general concepts. This process, which Glaser and Strauss call *"the method of constant comparison"*, is dedicated to the understanding, interpretation and interpretation of experiential data, and is translated as object-based theory building (cf. Breuer, 2010: 53ff).

The research style of Grounded Theory was developed in the 1960s by the American sociologists Barney Glaser and Anselm Strauss and later continued by Strauss and Juliet Corbin. Grounded theory is applied to disciplines of human action in sociology, psychology and pedagogy. Therefore, this research style is suitable when a deeper understanding of larger text sets is necessary, but also when new contexts and considerations as well as recommendations for action for a subject area are derived from the texts. Strauss and Corbin also recommend grounded theory to try out new ways of thinking about a problem area (cf. Strauss/Corbin, 1990: 12; quoted in: Bohm, 1994: 123).

This means that the aim of the work in grounded theory is usually field-specific. The aim is not to form universally valid theories and models, but a grounded theory developed on the basis of the data is always related to the phenomenon under investigation (cf. Bohm, 1994: 121).

The research logic of grounded theory is that all work steps run in parallel and influence each other productively. This means that through this parallelism of the work steps, statements can already be made and results produced with the analysis of the first case. Therefore, it makes sense to choose the first case to be analysed with care, as it has a great influence on the theory-building process.

Strauss and Corbin emphasise the factor of creativity in grounded theory. This includes a creative contribution by the researchers themselves, which is understood as a subjective contribution to the research process. To avoid subjective "surpluses", Strauss recommends organising research as a collective process in which researchers complement each other (cf. Strubing, 530-532; cited in Bauer/Blasius, 2018).

Thus, it is the task of the researcher to transform insights and incidents into relevant categories. These form the main source of all significant theorising (cf. Glaser/Strauss, 1998: 255ff).

The term "grounded theory" thus refers to the process and the results, as well as to a problem-free research action and the theories produced in the process. This means that grounded theory can be used to answer specific and predominantly research questions that have to do with an action or a process. Grounded theory is particularly suited to the study of phenomena where personal experience is important. The research question should provide the necessary flexibility and freedom to investigate a phenomenon in depth (cf. Strauss/Corbin, 1996: 22).

From the researcher's point of view, grounded theory is suitable for answering her research question for the reason that it is about the process of experiencing a nursing counselling interview in an oncological setting and its difficulties. Questions in grounded theory always have an action and process orientation (Strauss/Corbin, 1996: 23).

The perspective of the nurses, their reality and their experience during a nursing counselling interview with patients and their relatives in the oncological setting are the focus of this research work. The personal experiences of the staff members are subjective experiences from which insights for the nursing counselling interview in the oncological setting are gained.

3.3 Sampling and random sampling

This chapter is dedicated to the theoretical background of sampling in qualitative research. It also discusses how sampling and the selection of the sample are implemented in the present study.

3.3.1 Theoretical background of sampling and sampling design

In the research style of grounded theory, the sample is chosen in a process-accompanying manner, depending on the respective state of one's own development of knowledge and theory. This means that traps, variations and contrasts are selected that expand and enrich the knowledge about the object of investigation, but also secure and consolidate it. The theoretical knowledge achieved in each case is the basis for further decisions by the researcher. The sample size is relatively small because the collection and processing of qualitative data is very time-consuming and the focus is on the development and differentiation of theories (Breuer et al, 2009: 58).

According to Strauss, "*theoretical sensitivity*[1] refers to the researcher's qualifications. At the beginning of a research project, the competences are more or less pronounced and develop further during the engagement. An attitude of self-awareness, social attentiveness as well as linguistic accuracy and differentiation are advantageous. The demand and development of theoretical sensitivity can be done by the researchers through engagement with literature from different text genres. Ongoing self-reflection and reflection on topics, but also one's own professional experience, are prerequisites in dealing with the research material. (cf. Breuer et al., 2009: 59f).

The personal experiences and observations of the researcher in everyday nursing care show that staff members are afraid of unanswered questions during counselling. But also the lack of professional competence has an effect on the design of a nursing consultation and the relationship with the patient. The daily nursing routine also leaves little time for a detailed nursing consultation. The lack of standardised structures for professional nursing counselling leads to the fact that the staff members design the nursing counselling intuitively. These existing preconceptions lead the researcher to focus her attention on nursing counselling in the oncology setting. Referring to the hermeneutic circle, the researcher therefore assumes that professional counselling in nursing is only possible when the issues, obstacles and difficulties of the staff members in nursing counselling in the oncological setting are recognised and understood. Glaser and Strauss describe that the researcher has prior knowledge that comes from his/her personal experience, research experience and knowledge of the literature (cf. Strauss, 1998: 48).

The use of examples and occurrences, as well as events, actions and populations, which are guided by the developing theory, is called *theoretical sampling* and is used to make comparisons (cf. Strauss, 1998: 49).

Data collection or "*theoretical sampling*" is not planned in the medium or long term, but is based on relevant points in the research process. This means that certain concepts are significant for the researchers because they occur repeatedly in the comparison or do not appear at all. The aim is to select events and occurrences that are indicators of categories, their properties and dimensions (cf. Strauss/Corbin, 1998: 149; cf. Glaser/Strauss, 1998: 118).

The decision as to which data should be collected first and which direction the data collection should take can therefore not be planned (cf. Glaser/Strauss, 1998: 55).

Theoretical saturation" is achieved through meaningful data. The complete data does not reveal any other new concepts, categories, characteristics and dimensions. Due to the limited research time of this study within the framework of her qualification thesis, it is only possible for the researcher to derive a medium-range theory from the categories obtained after the conclusion of the data collection and data analysis.

3.3.2 Sampling and sample of the study

The question of which respondents should be included in the sample and why, as well as the description of the sampling process are defined in the following section.

The selection of the test persons for this study took place during the process. The researcher, in her role as a long-term ward manager of an oncology department, made a targeted selection of her staff members of the senior service for health care and nursing in the oncology setting of a primary care hospital, who had a wealth of experience and a broad spectrum of knowledge, but also subjects who had only gained little experience in the oncology setting. The researcher conducted the first interview with a staff member who has many years of professional experience and has completed further training in oncology in accordance with §64 GuKG. This is because she assumes that many years of professional experience and oncological training according to §64 GuKG will provide different information in the interview compared to a respondent with little professional experience. The researcher assumes that each case from the research field will contribute something to the theory of the subject. Holloway and Wheeler describe *purposive sampling* as the proposal to select a sample that deliberately selects/provides for people who have insight into the field of enquiry and can provide different information about the phenomenon under investigation (Holloway/Wheeler, 2010: 138).

The following table gives a detailed description of the test persons:

Interview partner/age	Expertjnnen	Additional training	Definition of the Additional training
IP 1/48a Pre-Test	DGKS	yes	Further training in complementary aroma nursing in accordance with Section 64 of the GuKG
IP2/46a	DGKS	yes	Further training in oncological nursing according to § 64 GuKG
IP 3/50a aborted	DGKS	no	
IP 4/23a	DGKS	no	
IP 5/30a	DGKS	no	
IP6/47a	DGKP	yes	Further training in oncological nursing according to § 64 GuKG
IP 7125a	DGKS	yes	Further training in practical guidance according to § 64 GuKG
IP 8/46a	DGKS	yes	Further training in pain management (Pain Nurse) according to §64 GuKG '

Table 1: Overview table of interview participants (age/job title/additional training/name of additional training)

The table shows that four out of six test persons have completed further training according to § 64 GukG. Two of the test persons have completed training in oncological nursing and one test person has completed training as a pain nurse. Furthermore, it is evident that not only older, experienced staff members of the higher service for health care and nursing have completed further training, but also one respondent with little experience in the oncological setting has already completed further training as a practice supervisor.

In the further procedure, the selected respondents were informed about the procedure of the study. All six interviews were scheduled between March and May 2019. The consent form for the interview was signed before the interview began. The researcher ensured that the interviews were transcribed and analysed in a timely manner. This enabled the validity of the resulting concepts to be tested for further interviews. This is in line with the theorising anchored in grounded theory. The researcher's field notes and observations of the subjects were included in the theory building.

3.4 Data collection

The first phase of the research process is to work out one's own pre-understanding and preconceptions about the subject area. Helpful methods are brainstorming and discussions in the group, but also reading relevant literature. The researcher of this study sketched out a mind-map in advance with the staff members of the higher service for health care and nursing, who did not participate in the study, in a lively exchange and with the help of these topics created the narrative guideline as support for the interview:

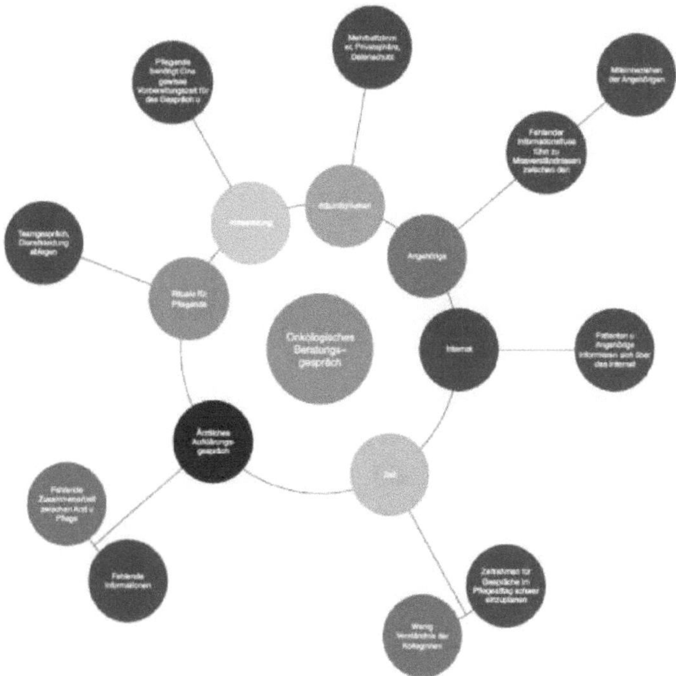

Figure 5: Mindmap (own representation)

The researcher of this study decided to conduct a narrative guided interview with six staff members of the senior health and nursing service in the oncology setting of a primary care hospital. Furthermore, an observation protocol is kept during the interviews. This includes observations of the test persons, but also the researcher's own state of mind during the interviews. In the context of the research, the researcher's daily cooperation in the ward's everyday life was another important access to the research field. Throughout the research process, notes were taken of conversations with ward staff who did not participate in the research.

3.4.1 The narrative guided interview

The interviews conducted by the researcher are described as narrative guided interviews, which were conducted face-to-face with six staff members of the senior health and nursing service in the oncology setting in a primary care hospital in Vorarlberg. The characteristics are closeness to everyday life, openness in terms of content and flexibility in the conduct of the interview, but also in the choice of topics.

The head of the nursing service and the head of the department as well as the six interviewees were informed in advance about the initial situation, the objectives and the procedure during the interview.

- Execution

Before the interviews, the written consent form was handed out to the respondents and they were given the opportunity to answer any questions that arose. They were also informed that they could end the interview at any time without giving a reason. The interviews began with a narrative prompt. The interviewees were asked to tell about certain situations and how they experience them. The atmosphere during the interviews was personal and coherent. A relaxed atmosphere eased the initial bias between the researcher and the respondent. The course of the interview was flexible in order to allow for a

to be able to ensure an uninterrupted flow of speech from the interviewees. The interview could be guided by maintenance questions and follow-up questions with thematic focal points, which the researcher used as a support tool for the interviews. This guide gave the researcher confidence at the beginning of the interviews, as some of the respondents felt a little uncertain at the start of the interviews and the narrative flow could thus be improved. The full version of the narrative guided interview can be found in the appendix.

The researcher conducted a pre-test interview with one respondent. The interview was conducted at the respondent's home, as the respondent was still uncertain about how to use the recording device and the supporting narrative interview guide. According to the respondent, he/she felt more relaxed in familiar surroundings. The dictation device and the recording function of the IPAD allowed for a problem-free recording and playback of the interview. The nervousness of the test person/proband could be recognised by the strong voice at the beginning of the interview. During the interview, the voice became normal and softer. The interview duration of 44 minutes in the pre-test showed that the concentration of the respondent and the researcher was lagging. This meant that the following interviews lasted between 16 to 35 minutes and the subjects were able to initiate the end themselves.

Two of the six interviews took place in empty patient rooms in the ward of the primary care hospital, as this was the least likely place to be disturbed by colleagues or other patients. Also, no unwanted telephone calls were possible in the rooms, which could interrupt the interview. The other four interviews were held in the office of the ward manager or the researcher. This in turn led to one respondent saying that she felt a little uncomfortable because it felt like an "examination". However, all respondents showed up for the pre-scheduled interview willingly and in a positive mood. After the interviews were completed, the next steps of the research were explained to the respondents.

- Transcription

The interviews were recorded and transcribed using a dictation machine and an IPAD. The transcription of the interviews began immediately after the first interview, so that the data analysis began parallel to the survey in the sense of a circular research process (cf. Strauss/Corbin, 1996: 8).

The transcription of the interviews was carried out by employees of the certified UniChamp GmbH in Vienna. The researcher decided to use simple transcription rules. The transcription was done in written German, the dialect was mostly smoothed. The everyday language, including faulty grammar, was retained and transcribed verbatim. The six interviews were pseudonymised and numbered IP 1-8. A total of eight interviews were conducted, one of which was used as a pre-test and another which was terminated and destroyed at the request of the respondent. The duration of the six interviews ranged from 16 to 35 minutes. The transcribed interview was handed out to all subjects.

3.4.2 The observation protocol during the interviews

An observation protocol was kept during the interviews. This includes observations of the test persons, but also the researcher's own state of mind during the interviews.

The researcher's observation record shows that during the interviews, four out of six subjects responded very well to the storytelling prompt. One interview was terminated at the request of the respondent. One respondent was very nervous during the whole interview. The researcher relates this to her simultaneous role as ward leader and researcher, which had an unsettling effect on the respondent. Furthermore, she could observe that at the beginning of the interview, the test persons were very deliberate and slow in their words, but after a short time, a fluent and relaxed course of conversation emerged. The subjects' voices were stronger, louder and nervous at the beginning, but during the course of the interview their tone and voice changed and they became calmer and more balanced. These observations were recorded in writing after each interview.

The following extract contains the documentation of observations made by the researcher during the interview:

IPS 46a	readily positive about IP	Interview takes place in the BuroderSL	Fluent in conversation. IP solution-oriented, empathetic, lack of training, shortage of doctors, multi-bed rooms, safety given.	Ended after 34 minutes, hardly any key topics completed - self-contained course of the conversation, interest in research results and transcript

Figure 6: Observation protocol - own representation (IP=interview partner/agreement/special features/conducted/after the interview)

All six respondents were positive and interested in the interview. The researcher was able to maintain eye contact with all the subjects during the interviews.

The researcher found the long pauses in the interviews irritating. The researcher also cites the fact that she intervened too quickly in the pauses during the first two interviews. The subsequent interviews could be conducted with more routine and confidence on the part of the interviewer.

3.4.3 Memos and diagrams

The course of the research process can be recorded in the form of memos and diagrams. Diagrams are graphic representations or visual images of relationships between concepts, while memos are the written form of abstract thinking of the data (cf. Strauss/Corbin, 1998: 169f).

Strauss/Corbin describe memos and diagrams as the product of inductive and deductive reasoning about categories and their properties and dimensions. Further, their relationships and variations, processes and the condition matrix (cf. Strauss/Corbin, 1998: 169).

Memos are reports that record progress but also pauses during a research process. This updates coding results and stimulates further coding processes so that a theory can be integrated. These written analysis protocols refer to the elaboration of the theory (cf. Strauss, 1998: 50; Strauss/Corbin 1998: 54).

In order to keep track of the texts during the analysis, it is helpful to write memos. The researcher uses theoretical memos for this study. They make it possible to recognise step-by-step interconnections. With the help of tables that were made to code the data, the first designations and overlaps could be documented. The defined concepts could thus be checked again and again for their meaningfulness. It was also necessary to rename the concepts several times and to make additions and deletions. For reasons of better readability, the memos used are only available to the researcher and are not cited in this paper.

3.5 Data analysis

The content of this chapter describes the method used to analyse the data. Each of the sub-chapters starts with a theoretical discussion of the methods and then moves on to their practical implementation, with theory and practice overlapping in places for ease of understanding.

3.5.1 Theoretical background of the coding methods

The analysis of the available data material is based on grounded theory. The theory to be developed should have as much stimulation as possible, only then is it possible to develop new paths of thought. Glaser supports researchers in this phase with his theoretical framework concepts that can be used for coding. These coding families contain a number of similar concepts. The coding families enable the researcher to reflect on and differentiate the research question. The principle of comparison in the evaluation process is to look for similarities and differences. The evaluation already starts with the first data collected. A concept will only find its way into the result of the study if it appears repeatedly in the documents studied. This means that it cannot be determined in advance what is to be examined in detail, but depends on the previous evaluation. It is therefore crucial for the researcher that the phenomenon is investigated in as many different contexts as possible, which allow for a wide range of comparisons (cf. Bohm, 1994: 124-126).

Through the cyclical repetition of coding and memo writing, as well as the purposeful collection of new data and engagement with existing data, new hypotheses are formed from the information and through the concepts and categories that emerge, the developing theory becomes denser and denser.

Strauss visualises the research process as follows:

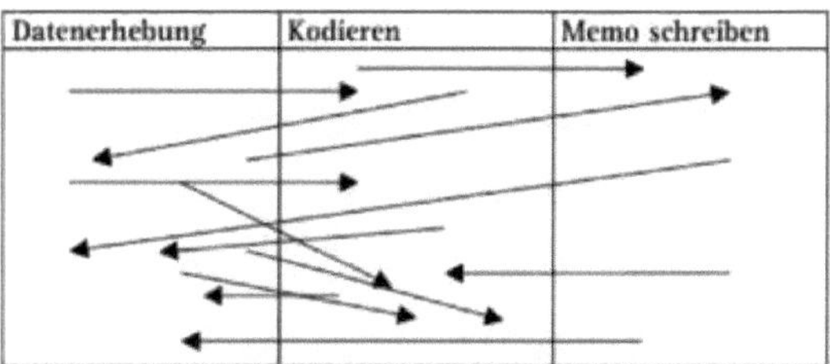

Figure 7: Research phases (cf. Strauss, 1994, n.d.)

Fundamental to the whole coding process is the concept-indicator model. Strauss describes this in that empirical indicators are concrete data, such as behaviours and events observed or described in interview texts, from which the researcher derives concepts. By comparing the indicators, categories are formed (cf. Strauss, 1998: 54).

3.5.2 Implementation of the data analysis

Theoretical coding is the central process of interpretation in grounded theory. "Code" is a term of the evaluation procedure and denotes a named concept. These preliminary concepts become more numerous and abstract in the course of the evaluation. Strauss already describes these differentiated concepts as categories. Coding means the analytical examination and development of text passages which are recognised as indicators of a concept. This results in lists of concepts and explanatory texts for the research process. In order to maintain an overview during the evaluation of the texts, it is helpful to write theoretical memos. In the course of the research process, hypotheses are developed as to how the categories can be linked to each other. Teamwork in the research process prevents one-sidedness and can accelerate the process of gaining knowledge (cf. Bohm, 1994: 124-126).

The researcher of this study sketched out a mind-map in advance with the staff members of the higher service for health care and nursing, who did not participate in the study, in a lively exchange and with the help of these topics she accelerated the research process and tried to reduce one-sidedness (see figure 5: mind-map).

3.5.3 Coding procedure

Coding is the term used to describe the process of analysis in grounded theory. The labelling of text passages refers to the whole process of analysis, the goal of which is theory building. Behind the process of analysis is the method of constant comparison. There is a constant interplay of selection, analysis and theory building. Consequently, coding means obtaining preliminary answers or hypotheses about categories and their interrelationships. The result of this analysis is a code that denotes a preliminary concept (cf. Strauss, 1998: 48).

This concept becomes more differentiated and abstract in the course of the evaluation, and is referred to as a category. Bohm describes coding as encoding or translating data, and it involves the naming and closer explanation of concepts (cf. Bohm, 2000: 476).

Strauss distinguishes three modes of coding and divides it into open, axial and selective coding (cf. Strubing, 2018: 535; cited in Bauer/Blasius, 2018).

3.5.3.1 Open coding

This is the analytical breaking down of data with the aim of conceptualising data and phenomena occurring in the text. Text passages are actively examined with supporting questions and marked with a code. These assigned codes can be used to search specifically for other text passages that contain similar or contrasting phenomena (cf. Strubing, 2018: 535; cited in Bauer/Blasius, 2018).

The interview with the test persons began with a narrative prompt: *"Please describe to me how you feel during a counselling session with your oncology patients and their relatives? How do you experience the relationship between relatives and patients? What situations come to your mind when you have conversations with patients and their relatives?*

The researcher uses the following example to show the steps of open coding in this research:

33-35	A...if you have any preparation now...how do you enter the conversation...?	Beginning of a counselling talk	
	IP4:... to pick up the patient where he is.	Empathising with the patient	
39-43	...the one is just in the exchange, the one is full of hate, the one is full of the why, in the fear, ...pick up, in the phase where he just is		Interpersonal Relationship building
	... which is quite bad for me, when now I'm		
44'45	there with my I go here, stand by the bed, rattle it off and go back.	Rational approach in the Counselling interview	Structure and process of a counselling interview
45-48	...first of all start a conversation and it's not about side effects, effects, ...but how has the Whole started,...	Hacking into prior knowledge of the Patients	Holism, humanistic Advisory concepts
51-52	... which I always think is great, to include relatives, because it's also a lot of information.	Dealing with relatives	Communication and interaction in care
53'55	... when emotions arise in a conversation, there is no right, no wrong, I decide that at that moment, I am simply inside that moment as a human being...		
	... Allowing emotions, supporting that,		
57-63	giving time,... I let it sink in and am quiet for a few seconds,...	Intuitive action with emotions	Self-care and resilience of

Figure 8: Example of open coding - own representation
(A=interviewer/IP=interviewee/wording/indicator/concept)

The example shows how the researcher derived indicators from the text passages and then defined the first concepts. A complete list of the concepts collected can be found in the appendix.

The background knowledge from the researcher's many years of professional experience is used in the open coding of the field under study to name the different aspects and characteristics of the phenomenon under study. For open coding, the search for in vivo codes is supportive, as they are colloquial interpretations of the phenomena from the direct field of study. Writing memos is helpful during the coding phases, as they are needed for the later structuring of the evaluation (see chapter 3.4.3). Traditional categories such as age, education and experience of the respondents are not yet relevant in open coding in this research. Organising these initial results already allows the researcher to see which concepts are important for the research question and need to be analysed in more depth.

Open Coding - Concepts	Interviewees (IP)
Proximity/Distance/Delimitation	IP2.4.6.8
Disease management in cancer	IP 2
Rituals at the end of a nursing counselling session	1Р2Л5Л8
Privacy and Intimacy through Physical Circumstances	IP 2, 4, 7, 8
Framework conditions of professional counselling	IP2,4,5,6,7,8
Counselling process	IP 5
Experiences, Experiences and	IP 2. 4. 5. 6. 7, 8
Communication disorders	IP 4. 5
Conflicts in communication with relatives	IP 5
Interpersonal relationship	IP 5
Counselling quality, counselling	IP 4. 5
Prior knowledge in the field of Communication/counselling in care	IP 7

Figure 9: Excerpt of concepts in open coding (own representation)

Through this assignment of codes, data become "indicators" and denote an underlying concept. By constantly comparing the codes, the theoretically relevant concepts are condensed. In a further coding step, these concepts become categories and result in a core category that can be related to all other categories that have been identified. This is called the concept-indicator model, which is based on the induction principle (Mey/Mruck, 2007: 25).

This leads to the next step in the coding process, "axial coding" (cf. Bohm, 1994: 128f).

3.5.3.2 Axial coding

Axial coding is used to refine and differentiate existing concepts that were formed during open coding. The researcher identified the following preliminary, central and significant categories based on the concepts that emerged during open coding:

- **Category 1**: *Near and far*

- **Category 2**: *Procedure and structure*

- **Category 3**: *Role and attitude*

- **Category 4**: *Prior knowledge*

The names of these preliminary categories are partly own designations, partly "in - vivo codes", these are terms and designations borrowed from the interviews (cf. Strauss/Corbin, 1996: 49f).

Each of the four main categories "*Proximity and Distance*", "*Process and Structure*", as well as "*Role and Attitude*" and "*Prior Knowledge*" have sub-categories, which in turn contain a number of sub-units, so-called dimensions. Existing subcategories are also related to each other. For a better understanding of the research results, the researcher gives examples and quotes from the data material of the interviews conducted.

Strauss/Corbin refer to the classification of concepts that are compared with each other and refer to a similar phenomenon as a category. This grouping of concepts is the basis of a category (cf. Strauss/Corbin, 1998: 43).

In the next step of axial coding, the researcher describes the relationships between a category and the formal and substantive aspects related to it, i.e. how the individual concepts are related to each other. Axial coding involves making comparisons by asking questions of the data (cf. Strauss/Corbin, 1996: 86).

- **Category 1: Closeness and distance in the nursing counselling interview**

How do carers deal with stress in oncological counselling sessions? What strategies do they use to relieve themselves? How do they distinguish themselves in counselling sessions? How do they deal with illness?

The following concepts refer to category 1:

- Near-dislance delimitation (IP2)
- Mental hygiene (IP2)
- Touch in care (IP2)
- Privacy and Intimacy in Spatial Circumstances (I P2)
- Framework conditions of professional guidance (IP2)
- Coping with cancer (IP2)
- Coping strategies of carers (I P2)
- Self-care and resilience of carers in the oncology setting (IP4)

- Near/Distance (IP4)
- Human images and values in the oncology setting (IP4)
- Self-care (IP4)
- At the end of the talk, shake hands, do a breath release ritual (IP4).
- Summarise conversation with teammate (IP5)
- Disease management (I P5)
- Proximity/Distance/Limitation (IP5)
- Coping strategies(IP5)
- Carers as a mouthpiece between patient/caregiverZAizt(IP5)
- SIE form in dealing with patientjn (IPS)
- Relationship and content level HOW/WHAT (Watzlawick) (IPS)
- Axiom of digital vs. analogue communication(S)
- Communication in Care (IPS)
- Client-centred approach Axioms 1-5) (IPS)
- Disease Management(IPS)
- Rituals of caregivers in the oncology setting after complex speech: (IPS)
- Self-care(IPS)
- Exchange with colleagues|(I PS)
- Rituals: Taking off uniforms(IPZ)

Figure 10: Concepts for the axial coding of the category *"proximity/distance"* (own representation)

The ordered and structured results of the open coding decide on the choice of the axial category for which further elaboration seems worthwhile. A detailed list of the open coding can be found in the appendix.

The researcher has defined three sub-categories *in the* previous category 1 *"Closeness and distance in nursing counselling* in *the oncology setting"*, which are called *person-centred communication, content and relationship level,* and *rituals, self-care and resilience.*

Concepts that pay into the subcategory of *person-centred communication*:

- Proximity/Distance/Delimitation
- Human images and values in the oncological setting
- SIE-form in dealing with the patient
- Client-centred approach - Axioms 1-5

Concepts which pay to the subcategory *content and relationship level*:

- Vocational training in care
- Privacy and intimacy through spatial circumstances
- Coping strategies
- Nurses as a mouthpiece between patients/caregivers/doctors
- Relationship and content level HOW/WHAT (Watzlawick)
- Axiom digital vs analogue communication
- Disease management in cancer

Concepts that pay into the subcategory of *rituals, self-care and resilience*:

- Mental hygiene
- Self-care and resilience of carers in the oncology setting
- Coping strategies of carers

- Communication in care
- At the end of the talk shake hands, take a puff - release ritual
- Summarise with teammates
- Exchange with colleagues
- Ritual - Removal of uniforms

After this careful sorting of the concepts for category 1 *"Closeness and distance in nursing counselling in the oncological setting"* in the subcategory *person-centred communication*, the researcher comes to the conclusion that nurses use the word YOU in their form of address when dealing with patients and their relatives because it helps them to maintain an appropriate relationship between closeness and distance and the associated demarcation in the nursing counselling conversation:

"The SIE form,...even if someone says you to me, especially the oncological patients who come again and again,...you actually always create distance for yourself (IP6: 253)."

The nurses' images of humanity and values in the oncological setting, as well as their own approach to illness and health, determine whether they stand apart from or are close to the patients:

".who are your age,...have similar interests and are still fully in life,.then it is more difficult (IP6: 255-269)."

In the subcategory *content and relationship level, it* becomes apparent that a relationship with the patients can only be established if privacy and intimacy are made possible by the spatial conditions:

".one of the difficulties I see is when you have to do it in a four-bed room now (IP2:10-15)."

The decisive factor in communication between carers and patients is HOW and WHAT is said, so that a trusting relationship is established:

"Allowing emotions, supporting that, giving time,...I let it sink in and be quiet for a few seconds (IP4: 57-63)."

In the subcategory *rituals, self-care and resilience,* the exchange of team colleagues before and after a nursing consultation is important. The subsequent reflection in the team helps the staff to cope with difficult situations in the next discussion. Rituals are used after stressful nursing consultations:

"... that I can leave that behind when I go out of the house, as soon as I take off my work clothes (IP7: 143-145)."

This results in the following assumption for the researcher in category 1 *Closeness and distance in the nursing consultation in the oncological setting*: The younger the patients to be cared for in the nursing consultation in the oncological setting, the more difficult it is for the nurses to distance themselves.

- **Category 2: Structure and process of a nursing consultation in the oncology setting**

What is the process of a nursing consultation in an oncology setting? What help do nurses need to conduct a professional nursing consultation? What framework conditions are necessary?

In the previous category 2 *"Structure and process of a nursing counselling session in the oncological setting"*, three subcategories were defined, which are referred to as the *framework conditions of a nursing counselling* session, the counselling *process* and the *counselling approaches.* A detailed list of the concepts can be found in the appendix.

Concepts which pay to *the* subcategory *framework conditions of nursing counselling*:

- Psychosocial services, psychooncology
- Privacy and intimacy through spatial circumstances
- Networking in counselling by carers

Concepts that pay into the subcategory of *guidance process*:

- Preparation of the conversation
- Define contents: Therapy, side effects, cycle, open questions result in different procedure
- Relationship building
- Documentation in nursing counselling

Concepts that fall into the subcategory of *guidance approaches*:

- Integrative guidance process: naming/experiencing/reflecting/rehearsing

After careful sorting, the researcher found in the previous category 2 *"Structure and procedure of a nursing counselling session in the oncological setting"* in the subcategory *framework conditions* that multiprofessional cooperation with psychosocial services, but also a network of contact partners, belong to the necessary structures of a nursing counselling session. In order to ensure an uninterrupted process of a nursing counselling session, a privacy-creating and confidential environment in a suitable room on the ward is required.

"...and also have the peace, okay the bell can be ringing now, that's not so tragic...or space, because the fewer interruptions, the more fluently the conversation runs (IP5: 268-274)."

The subcategory *consultation process* shows that the preparation of the nursing consultations takes a lot of time for the nurses and that there is a lack of rooms in which an undisturbed preparation can take place. The preparation is further dependent on whether the nurses were already able to be present at the medical consultation. This is because important information about the treatment and the course of the disease is already helpful for the nurses in the further consultation, and thus supports the relationship between the participants. The main contents of a nursing consultation refer to the process and side effects of chemotherapy, as well as to questions that the patients and their relatives have already researched on the internet and bring with them:

".especially in times of the internet, people are very enlightened, partly misinformed and the misinformation has to be cleared out of the way.modern forms of therapy cannot yet be distinguished by lay people (IP6: 47-58)".

Furthermore, the nurses state that incomplete documentation of nursing consultations makes the further course of a conversation more difficult. This is because it is not always possible to include all the contents in the first consultation.

In the sub-category counselling *approaches, it* can be seen that the nurses compare the nursing counselling interview with the medical clarification interview, in that they mainly concentrate on the medical focal points in the counselling.

This leads to the following assumption for the researcher in category 2 *Structure and process in the nursing counselling interview in the oncological setting*: The more information the nurses receive before a nursing counselling interview, the more precisely the disease process and treatment plan are discussed and the more privacy can be maintained during a counselling interview, the more confident and competent the nurses feel in the nursing counselling.

- **Category 3: The role and attitude of carers and relatives in the oncological counselling interview**

What is the relationship of the carers to the patients? What is the relationship between carers and relatives? What role does the doctor-caregiver relationship play?

In the previous category 3 *"Role and attitude in the oncological counselling interview"* three subcategories were defined, which were called *"The role of the nurse, the role of the relatives and the doctor-nurse relationship"*. A detailed list of the concepts can be found in the appendix.

Concepts that pay to the subcategory *The role of nurses in the oncology counselling interview:*

- Active listening - paraphrasing
- Communication with seriously ill patients

- Verbal, non-verbal and para-verbal communication
- Communication and interaction in care
- Empathy, congruence and acceptance (according to Rogers)

Concepts that pay attention to the subcategory *role of relatives in oncology counselling:*

- Conflicts in communication with relatives
- Involvement of relatives
- Interpersonal relationship

Concepts that pay to the *doctor-nurse relationship* subcategory:

- Reflection of the discussions, teamwork
- Patient-centred communication
- Quality of the counselling

After careful sorting, the researcher found in the previous category 3 in the subcategory *The role of nurses in oncology counselling* that patient compliance and self-determination depend on the extent to which nurses bring genuineness and acceptance as well as empathy to the counselling. Communication and interaction are crucial for the quality of the nurses' counselling. In difficult conversations and situations, this depends on the personal experiences, experiences and feelings of the carers:

..... Trust is important and what you actually bring to the patient unconsciously every day, you have to bring within a few minutes,... professional, human, trust (IP4: 192-194)."

The central basis of the nurse is the encounter with the patient, which includes the physical and psychosocial level. This theory of care corresponds to the ideas of the philosophy of holism. A core principle of holism *is "the whole is more than the sum of its parts"* and thus defines the unity of body, mind and spirit in the care of patients and their relatives.

In the subcategory The *role of relatives in oncological counselling*, it is shown that carers perceive relatives as a burden. The defensive attitude towards them makes it difficult to build up interpersonal relationships. Conflicts in communication with relatives arise from a one-sided relationship between the nurses and the patients and thus exclude the relatives.

What I find difficult is when patients and relatives are anxious, have a lot of questions, when you have a conversation where you can't finish, where questions keep coming. ...when relatives make the patient feel insecure themselves (IP4: 171-174)".

In the subcategory *doctor-nurse-relationship,* it is shown that the quality of the nursing consultation depends on whether nurses were already able to be present during the doctor's explanatory consultation. The cooperation between nursing and doctor also determines the main content of a nursing consultation as well as the relationship to the patients and their relatives, since an interpersonal relationship already develops during the doctor's consultation. The importance of the nursing consultation thus increases if the nurses can already be present during the doctor's consultation.

This leads to the following assumption for the researcher in the preliminary category 3 *Role and attitude of nurses and relatives in nursing counselling in the oncological setting:* The more professional experience nurses have in nursing counselling, the better they can empathise with and understand the patients and their relatives. The less experience nurses have in nursing counselling, the more they are dependent on information from a doctor's clarification interview so that an interpersonal relationship with trust, empathy and acceptance can develop between the patients and their relatives.

- **Category 4: Prior knowledge in nursing counselling in the oncology setting**

What previous knowledge and experience do nurses have in nursing counselling? In the previous category 4 "*Prior knowledge in nursing counselling in the oncology setting*", two subcategories were defined, which are referred to as *legal basis* and *counselling quality*. A detailed list of the concepts can be found in the appendix.

Concepts that pay into the subcategory of *legal foundations*:

- Knowledge enhancement
- Education, training and continuing education in oncological care
- Expertise for professional counselling in care
- Counselling training in care, legal basis
- Patient charter and legal basis
- Nursing Core Competencies/Multiprofessional Competency Area (§64 GukG)

Concepts that pay into the subcategory of *quality of guidance*:

- Professional experience
- Intelligible language in patient communication
- Support from superiors
- Previous knowledge and experience
- Counselling deficits
- Professional competences
- Internet
- Coherence: comprehensibility, manageability, meaningfulness are goals of guidance
- Competencies

After careful sorting, the researcher finds in the previous category 4 "*Prior knowledge*" that in the subcategory *Legal foundations,* further training in oncological nursing (according to §64 GukG) does not significantly increase the specialist knowledge for professional nursing counselling. Also the existence of theoretical knowledge from the training for the higher service for health care and nursing is only helpful in practice after personal experience:

..... So at school you can never really put yourself in the situation as it really is on the ward,...it only really comes when you do it yourself (IP7: 176-178)".

Nurses assume that medical knowledge about the treatment plan and the course of the disease will improve their competence in counselling, and thus the quality of counselling.

In the subcategory *quality of counselling,* it is shown that younger staff members have more counselling deficits and that the quality of counselling thus depends on the professional experience and previous knowledge of the nurses:

Yes, when questions keep coming in detail, that challenges me, when you don't really get a chance to talk things out, you keep getting interrupted and asked very critical questions (IP7: 60-62)".

The goals of nursing counselling, which include comprehensibility, manageability and meaningfulness, depend on the core nursing competencies of the nurses, which thus define the quality of counselling.

Furthermore, the internet knowledge of the patients and their relatives influences the quality of the counselling provided by the nurses. The challenges are that questions and uncertainties can be discussed with the patients and their relatives in an understandable language.

...an older patient who is not an Internet type now,...naturally needs a different explanation than someone who has googled a lot and has already informed himself very well in advance,...that is noticeable that people are very well informed (IP6: 99-105)."

This leads to the following assumption for the researcher in the preliminary category 4 *Prior knowledge in nursing counselling in the oncological setting*: The less communicative competences are available in nursing counselling, the greater the fear of nurses of not being able to answer unforeseen questions, and the more support nurses need from their superiors to improve their counselling deficits in the form of training and further education.

The following step describes the process of "relating" in axial coding.

One of the central aspects of axial coding is also the "relating" of categories. Here, text passages are coded further and new codes are formulated or existing ones are used so that relations between the axial categories and other codes can be determined. Individual passages are interpreted "axially", but also several passages are compared and interpreted. This procedure is similar to open coding, but the decisive step in axial coding is to work out relationships between the axial categories and the concepts related to them in the content and formal aspects. Relationships in axial coding refer to temporal and spatial relationships of the axial category, cause-effect relationships also count. In addition to means-purpose relationships, argumentative and motivational relationships are important in axial elaboration. In axial coding, hypotheses are tested on the basis of new data material, so that it finally leads to a plausibility check.

These hypotheses represent a preliminary answer to a question about the concepts, about the phenomenon and about the relationship of different phenomena to each other. These connections of the relationships and the categories thus form a section of the object-anchored theory (cf. Strauss/Corbin, 1998: 44).

- **Hypothesis Category 1: Proximity and distance**

The younger the patients to be cared for in the nursing consultation in the oncological setting, the more difficult it is for the nurses to distinguish themselves.

- **Hypothesis Category 2: Procedure and structure**

The more information the nurses receive before a nursing consultation, the more precisely the course of the disease and the planned treatment plan are discussed and the more privacy can be maintained during a consultation, the more confident and competent the nurses feel in the nursing consultation.

- **Hypothesis Category 3: Role and attitude of carers and relatives and doctor-nurse relationship**

The more professional experience nurses have in nursing counselling, the better they can empathise with and understand patients and their families. The less experience nurses have in nursing counselling, the more they need information from a doctor's exploratory talk to establish an interpersonal relationship with trust, empathy and acceptance between the patients and their relatives.

- **Hypothesis Category 4: Prior knowledge**

The less communication skills are available in nursing counselling, the greater is the fear of nurses not being able to answer unforeseen questions, and the more support nurses need from their superiors to improve their counselling deficits in the form of education and training.

Strauss and Corbin developed a coding paradigm for the elaboration. With the help of this search heuristic, categories are created according to the conditions, the interaction

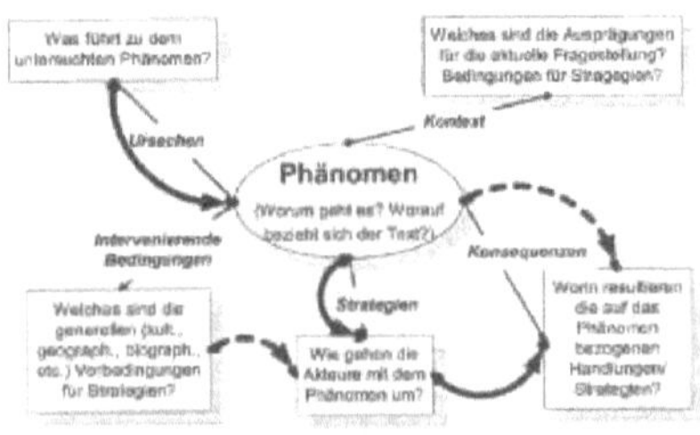

Abbildung11: Coding paradigm (Strubing, 2008: 28)

At the centre of axial coding is the *phenomenon*. Every phenomenon has a *cause*. The persons acting in the research field deal with the phenomenon in a certain way. This is called a *strategy*. An implemented strategy consequently has *consequences,* such as events and happenings. Strauss and Corbin relate the *context* to the phenomenon. The *intervening conditions* are called structural conditions that influence actions and interactions (cf. Strauss/Corbin, 1998: 75f).

The aim of axial coding is to work out the categories that are necessary for theory building. In addition, the relationships between the axial categories and their individual subcategories are worked out. A linkage between the main categories leads to further results in the presentation (cf. Flick, 2007: 393).

3.5.3.3 Selective Coding

The axis categories found are classified again until a core category emerges. This is then briefly described together with its relationships, which is referred to in English as the story. The theory is then formulated and re-examined on the basis of the data (cf. Flick 2007: 396).

For the researcher, in-depth axial coding is sufficient for answering the specific research question, as this is how she arrived at a conclusive coding paradigm, which is described in the presentation of results (cf. chapter 4). Selective coding" is therefore - within the framework of the "presentation of results" - only hinted at or further questions are also posed for which selective coding would be appropriate in order to be able to answer these new and further research questions.

3.6 Good criteria of qualitative research

The core criteria that relate to qualitative social research include documenting the research process. In this research, the researcher has recorded all the steps of the process, and extracts of them are presented in this paper in the form of lists and tables. For the interpretation, the researcher had already had a lively exchange with the staff members of the upper-level service for health care and nursing before the beginning of the research, and outlined this with the help of a mind map (see figure: 5). This was done so that the criteria of interpretation in groups could be fulfilled to some extent. A codified procedure was used. The researcher of this thesis decided on a qualitative research approach due to the research question in order to gain an insight into topics in the context of a nursing counselling interview of the staff of the higher service for health care and nursing in the oncological setting. In order to develop an object-related theory in this research work, grounded theory is used within the framework of qualitative research. The steps of the research include codified methods and textual evidence, as well as the use of analytical induction, inferable and testable predictions, and communicative validation. The limitations of the research are stated in the Limitation (see Chapter 6: Outlook and Limitations). The research topic of this study is considered relevant by the researcher. This is shown by the fact that there was already a great interest in the interviews of the staff of the higher service for health care and nursing in the oncological setting, and with the research topic it is described in detail that nursing counselling competences are of essential importance in the oncological setting. Reflective subjectivity was established through self-observation by the researcher during the

interviews. As they work directly with the respondents in the research field, there is a familiar and open relationship between them (cf. Steinke, 2000; cited in Breuer et.al., 2009: 109-110).

4 Presentation of the results

In the following section, the preliminary results of the axial coding are presented. For the researcher, a more in-depth axial coding is sufficient to answer the specific research question, as it enabled her to arrive at a conclusive coding paradigm. In the first section, the four surveyed categories *"closeness and distance"*, *"set-up and structure"*, *"role and attitude of the nurse/caregiver/physician/nurse relationship"*, and *"prior knowledge"* in the nursing counselling interview in an oncological setting are presented. In the second section, the results of the research question are presented according to the coding paradigm of the grounded theory methodology (cf. Figure 10).

4.1 Results of the axial coding

The connections and differences between the individual (sub)categories were elaborated in the process of axial coding. For a better understanding of the research results, the researcher gives examples and quotes from the data material of the interviews conducted.

The following graphical representation provides an overview of the four categories formed with the respective subcategories:

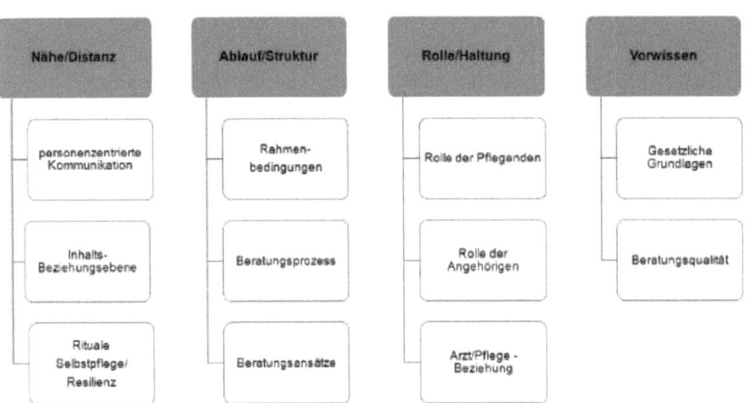

Table 2: Axial category formation (own representation)

4.1.1 Category 1 - Close and Distance

The category of closeness and distance was divided into three subcategories, which include *patient-centred communication, content and relationship levels, as well as rituals, self-care and resilience.*

With reference to the subcategory *patient-centred communication, it* is evident that all

"

six nurses make demarcation and the associated distance in the nursing consultation dependent on the age of the patients. Younger patients or patients of the same age are perceived as stressful by the nurses. One nurse describes that the patients' children represent an additional burden because she identifies with her own role as a mother:

"Bad situation, young patient, ... the age is quite telling, which then already concerns me, also when children are involved, ... which is not so easy...(IP5: 227-237). "

In counselling, the focus is not only on nursing expertise, but on understanding and appreciating the patients and their relatives in the respective situation, so that a professional relationship can be established. The basic attitude in counselling includes positive appreciation, authenticity and unconditional acceptance in the client-centred approach according to Carl Rogers. This means that patients are recognised as persons with their own values and their individuality is respected. The inner thinking and feeling of the nurses in counselling are the prerequisite for an empathic and appreciative congruence between nurses and patients (cf. Elzer/Sciborski, 2007: 84f).

In the subcategory *content and relationship level, it* is evident that younger nurses describe more fears about existential questions in conversation. It is also evident that younger nurses assume that their professional medical competences are decisive in the conversation, so that they can convey security and trust:

.....what I liked to do is to give the patient confidence, ...that I am competent with what I am doing and that they can feel confident about what I am giving them (IP6: 99-105)".

The communication scientist Paul Watzlawick bases his communication theory on five axioms, which state that communication always has an effect on the behaviour of patients and counsellors in care. Communication is divided into a content aspect (WHAT) and a relationship aspect (HOW). The predominantly verbal content aspect comprises factual information, in contrast to the verbal and non-verbal relationship aspect, which specifies how this information is to be understood by the receiver and how the sending person defines the relationship between him/herself and the receiving person. This means that if the interlocutors have a stable relationship, different opinions can be allowed without the relationship suffering or breaking down. The prerequisite is positive and appreciative interaction (cf. Watzlawick, 2016: 16).

On the other hand, nurses with many years of professional experience consider available space and the necessary privacy in conversation to be necessary for relationship building:

"What is important for me is when there is a bit of privacy,....(IP2:10)."

In addition to demanding competences through targeted education, training and further education as well as through reflected professional practice, the necessary working conditions for shaping a guidance process must also be supported.

In the subcategory *rituals, self-care and resilience,* five out of six nurses use rituals after stressful nursing counselling sessions:

"... and what for me is the real letting go afterwards - the shower, as if I were doing the washing up at home (IP4: 216)".

All six nurses use the exchange with their team colleagues before and after a nursing consultation:

"...if I get stuck, I can ask my team....can get someone and that gives me a good confidence even if a situation is not so easy (IP2: 193-202)".
Rituals after stressful conversations support and challenge the resilience of carers in the oncology setting.

4.1.2 Category 2 - Procedure and structure

The category of *process and structure* in nursing counselling is divided into three subcategories, which are defined as *framework conditions*, counselling *process* and *counselling approaches.*

In the sub-category of *framework conditions*, all six respondents complained that shared rooms hardly or not at all allow for privacy and intimacy in nursing consultations.

..... simply has a way to withdraw with the relatives and patients (IP7: 163-165)."
Furthermore, it can be seen that only one nurse states that she plans the nursing consultation with the patients and their relatives and arranges a joint appointment in advance.

The term "guidance" is a familiar form of communication used in everyday life, which is to be distinguished from professional guidance. Nestmann defines guidance as professional support that attempts to discover, challenge and maintain social relationships and networks, organisations and institutions as well as built and natural environments in a joint process of orientation, planning, decision-making and action (cf. Nestmann, 1997: 33-34).

In the subcategory *counselling process, it is* evident that younger nurses invest more time in the preparation of a nursing counselling session, as they make their own professional competences dependent on whether patients can trust them and whether they appear competent enough:

Preparation is important for me, that I simply have the feeling of security and simply also competence, that I can clarify the patient (IP 4: 16-18)".

In contrast, nurses with several years of professional experience design their counselling sessions intuitively:

"When people say, yes, I already know this and that, I'm only interested in this,...only respond to what they really ask.... or when you notice that they are overwhelmed,...that I notice that nothing more gets through (IP2: 144-154)."

Four out of six nurses state that the key points they have prepared must be fulfilled in the nursing consultation so that they have a positive feeling at the end of a conversation. For all six nurses, the structures and essential contents for a nursing consultation depend on the patient's cancer disease, the therapy and the side effects that will occur during the course of the disease. All six nurses concentrate in their preparation on the medical aspects of counselling. Although two of the nurses have completed further training in oncological nursing according to § 64, no preparations are made on how a consultation should be started or ended, and what happens if a patient breaks off the consultation.

In principle, counselling is process-oriented. This means that nurses in the oncology setting are able to respond directly to common difficulties. However, any professional conversation in the oncology setting requires planning of external and internal factors (cf. Baumer, 2008: 343).

Five out of six nurses lack involvement in the medical consultation with patients, relatives and the doctor in charge.

The multiprofessional area of competence in § 16 (3) of the higher service for health care and nursing includes nursing expertise in interprofessional networking, information transfer and knowledge management as well as the coordination of the treatment and care process, including ensuring the continuity of treatment (GuKG, version of 25.05.2019).

A lack of and incomplete documentation of the nursing counselling talks is cited by three nurses as a complication of recurrent counselling.

Carers often do not perceive the activity of counselling as a continuous task. As a result, counselling activities are not documented and thus not considered professional care activities (cf. Huper/Hellige, 2007: 102).

In the subcategory *counselling approaches, it is* evident that all six nurses use the term "clarification talk" for the nursing counselling talk in the oncology setting.

Nurses associate counselling with the communication of information and factual content, but in the context of nursing, counselling is also described as a relationship process between nurses, patients and their relatives (cf. Hummel-Gatz/Doll, 2007: n.d.).

4.1.3 Category 3 - Role and attitude

The category of *role and attitude of* the carer/relative and doctor/nurse relationship was divided into three subcategories, which were defined *as role and attitude of the carer, role* and *attitude of* the *relative* and *doctor/nurse relationship.*

In the subcategory *role and attitude of the nurses* in the oncological counselling discussion, it is shown that the compliance and self-determination of the patients depend on the extent to which the nurses can bring authenticity and acceptance as well as empathy into the counselling:

.....what I liked is to give the patient confidence, ...that I am competent with what I am doing and that they can feel confident about what I am giving them (IP 6: 99-105)."

This, in turn, depends on the personal experiences, experiences and feelings of the carer. The basic attitude of counselling according to Karl Rogers is characterised by an empathic, non-possessive warmth, sympathy and acceptance. This is how Newman describes the role of the carer as a life counsellor. This form of counselling involves more than informing, guiding and giving advice. The concept of counselling in Neumann's and Newman's theories includes psychosocial counselling competences, i.e. activities that do not belong to the nursing-specific competences (cf. Schaeffer et al. 1997: 251; quoted in Koch-Straube, 2008: 27f).

Younger nurses find it important that all relevant points are included in the nursing consultation, and they become unsettled as soon as they are interrupted by unexpected questions from patients and their relatives. Four carers find it important to recognise the needs in the nursing consultation:

"...Young women have different needs than perhaps older men, it's quite individual...(IP5:41)."

In order to explore the importance of communication and the relationship between patients, their relatives and carers, it is important to look at the principles of nursing theories. In a needs-based nursing theory, nurses support patients with the aim of regaining independence and performing the activities of daily living. This leads to considering self-realisation, self-responsibility and autonomy as the outcome of care, not taking into account the patient's personal potential (cf. Abdallah, Henderson, zin. In Koch-Straube, 2008: 21f).

In the subcategory *role and attitude of relatives*, four out of six carers state that they perceive relatives as a burden during a counselling session. One carer states that she would therefore like more time in the daily care routine to get to know the relatives:

"If you really take your time, you get statements or information where you often didn't know for a long time or where it suddenly makes sense that they act this way (IP4: 115-121).

Conflicts in communication with relatives arise from a one-sided relationship between the nurses and the patients, and thus exclude the relatives. The defensive attitude of the carers towards the relatives makes it difficult to build up interpersonal relationships.

In an outcome-oriented theory of care, the focus is not on creating a relationship between equal partners. This means that differentiated perspectives, the autonomy and obstinacy of patients and their relatives do not receive any recognition. For a concept of counselling, however, it is necessary that the individuality and subjective views of the patients and relatives are included (cf. Koch-Straube, 2008: 24).

In the subcategory *doctor-nurse-relationship* it becomes apparent that the quality of the nursing consultation depends on whether nurses were already able to be present during the doctor's explanatory talk. The cooperation between nursing and doctor also determines the main content of a nursing consultation and the relationship with the patients and their relatives, since an interpersonal relationship already develops during the doctor's consultation. The importance of their nursing consultation thus increases for the nurses if they can already be present during the doctor's consultation.

Ideally, a member of the senior health and nursing staff should also be present at a doctor's consultation. When delivering a diagnosis, honesty and trust between the doctor and the person concerned is a prerequisite to reduce fears. False hopes should be avoided in this discussion so that the patients and their relatives can make a realistic decision for the future (cf. Langkafel/Lucke, 2008: 42f).

4.1.4 Prior knowledge

In category 4 *Prior knowledge* in nursing counselling, two subcategories were defined, which are referred to as *Legal basis* and *Counselling quality*.

In the subcategory *legal basis*, four out of six nurses have completed further training according to §64 GuKG.

"we had a day.... situations based on a case study, role play, on oncological situations, where each patient was a doctor and had to pass on a diagnosis (IP7: 176)".

Nevertheless, all six nurses assume that medical knowledge about the treatment plan and the course of the disease improves their competences in counselling, and thus the quality of counselling, and not their communicative competences.

In the subcategory *quality of counselling,* it is shown that younger staff members have more counselling deficits and that the quality of counselling thus depends on the professional experience and previous knowledge of the nurses:

"Yes, when questions keep coming in detail,...that challenges me, when you don't really get a chance to talk things out, are interrupted again and again and are asked quite critically (IP7: 60-62)."

Human communication is influenced in terms of content and form by the psychological characteristics of the persons involved. Friedemann Schulz von Thun describes eight different communication styles that correlate with specific personality traits. These communication styles show possible communication disturbances, as they reveal typical sequences of relationship dynamics that can result in a disrupted course of conversation (cf. Elzer/Sciborski, 2007: 156).

Also, having theoretical knowledge of difficult languages is only helpful in practice after personal experience:

"So at school you can never really put yourself in the situation of what it's really like on the ward afterwards. It only really comes when you do it yourself (IP7: 177-178).

The goals of nursing counselling, which include comprehensibility, manageability and meaningfulness, depend on the core nursing competencies of the nurses and thus define the quality of counselling.

One nurse states that the existing internet knowledge of the patients and their relatives exerts a high pressure of expectation in the nursing consultation:

"That can also lead in the wrong direction, create fears, especially experiences. It's just what you then also get, the positive less on the internet, that's the dangerous thing, you have to point it out to people right away (IP6: 102-115)".

The challenges for three nurses are to be able to discuss questions and uncertainties that arise in an understandable language with patients and their relatives. Four out of six nurses assume that their expertise lies in being able to answer all questions, as this conveys confidence and security.

Gores writes that nurses must be able to acquire and apply communicative, interpretative, strategic and problem-solving competencies in addition to action competencies (cf. Elzer/Sciborski, 2007:103).

In client-centred counselling, Rogers defines active listening and paraphrasing as a technical form of intervention in leading the conversation. The repetition of the most important thoughts and feelings by the counsellors is defined as paraphrasing or mirroring of one's own performances. The counsellors' addressing of non-verbal behaviour as well as asking questions in case of ambiguities complete the guided conversation. Silence and pauses are also important components of a counselling conversation (cf. Elzer/Sciborkski, 2007: 86-87).

4.2 Presentation of results - Coding paradigm

To answer the research question, the researcher uses the coding paradigm (cf. chapter 3.5.3.2 Axial Coding). The focus is on the nursing consultation in the oncological setting of a primary care hospital in Vorarlberg. In this section, the researcher describes the initial conditions of a nursing counselling interview, the context of the counselling interview in the oncological setting, as well as the strategies of action used by the nurses and the resulting consequences.

4.2.1 Phenomenon - The nursing counselling interview in the oncological setting

Interaction and communication is a central part of counselling. In expert counselling, specialised nurses provide their knowledge and experience. This expert counselling takes place in the oncological setting between the patients, their relatives and the staff of the higher service for health care and nursing within the framework of a nursing counselling discussion.

The counselling process is often dynamic, because the individual phases overlap, but also merge or repeat. Engel describes the counselling process as a goal-oriented method of analysing, planning, implementing and reviewing, which is carried out together with the patient in the form of a dialogue, similar to the nursing process (cf. Engel, 2006: 49).

In this process counselling, the nurse sees him/herself as a supporter and challenger of a pending development during the disease process. Nurses are often the first contact persons for patients after the diagnosis of cancer. A close relationship develops between nurses and patients, but also with their relatives. These reactions of *not wanting to admit, only understanding in part* or not *hearing the most* or *immediately forgetting* lead to misunderstandings in the communication between those affected, doctors and nurses (cf. Weyland, 2013: 51).

The researcher of this study has therefore addressed the following question:

How do staff members of the higher service for health care and nursing experience the nursing counselling interview with patients and their relatives in the oncological setting of a primary care hospital in Vorarlberg?

For the researcher, in-depth axial coding is sufficient to answer the specific research question, as it has enabled her to arrive at a conclusive coding paradigm. Selective coding" is therefore only hinted at or further questions are posed for which selective coding would be appropriate in order to be able to answer these new and further research questions.

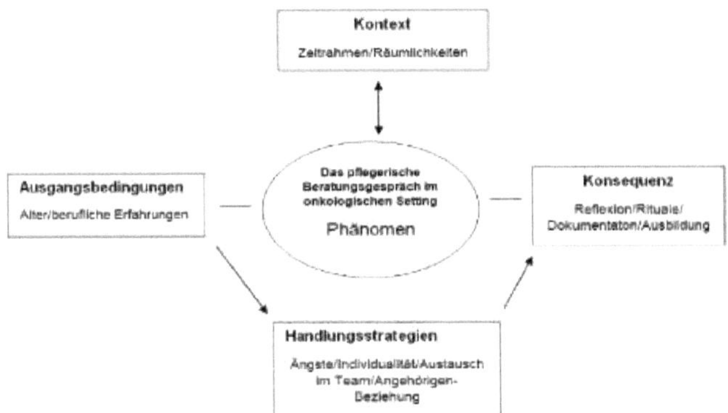

Figure 12: Coding paradigm (own representation)

4.2.2 The initial conditions

In principle, counselling is process-oriented. This means that nurses are able to respond directly to difficulties that are common among patients. However, any professional conversation in the oncological setting requires planning of external and internal factors for the communication process (cf. Baumer, 2008: 343).

The baseline conditions for a nursing counselling interview in the oncology setting in this study revealed that nurses make the following distinctions:

- **The age of the patients**

The nurses distinguish between younger and older patients. This is because they assume that younger patients will ask more and more detailed questions during the interview. Also because the nurses recognise themselves more in patients of the same age or younger. It is also recognisable that experienced nurses identify more strongly with patients who still have small children as relatives and are therefore less able to distinguish themselves.

The inner thinking and feeling of the carers is therefore the prerequisite for an empathic and appreciative congruence between carers and patients (cf. Elzer/Sciborski, 2007: 84f).

- **Professional experience in dealing with oncological patients**

Furthermore, it can be seen that younger inexperienced nurses invest more time in the preparation of a nursing counselling session, as they assume that they appear trustworthy and competent due to their medical expertise. Nurses assume that medical knowledge about the treatment plan and the course of the disease improves their competences in counselling, and thus the quality of counselling. On the other hand, professionally experienced staff members of the higher service for health care and nursing need hardly any time for the preparation of a nursing counselling interview. They design their contents and main topics individually and adapt them to the respective situation by asking the patients and their relatives about their previous knowledge.

In order to be able to offer counselling, nurses must expand their professional competences. The prerequisites for successful counselling in nursing are knowledge of the theoretical foundations of counselling and methodological competence, so that the counselling process can be designed in a goal-oriented and systematic way. But also the ability to perceive the patients and their relatives individually and the willingness to develop oneself further and to use oneself to understand situations are components of competences in counselling (cf. Koch-Straube, 2008: 182).

4.2.3 The context

In order for nursing counselling to be carried out in an oncological setting, the framework conditions and the agreement between the participants are the prerequisite for a helping relationship to develop. The setting influences the quality and limits of a conversation (cf. Elzer/Sciborski, 2007: 123).

From the collected data of the survey, the following results emerged for the staff of the higher service for health care and nursing:

- **Timeframe for preparation and implementation**

How long a nursing counselling interview lasts and which contents and main topics are addressed is decided by the staff members by already dealing with it during the preparation. For the preparation of a nursing counselling interview, the staff members of the higher service for health care and nursing with little or hardly any professional experience need more time. If it is an initial consultation with patients and their relatives, the nurses prepare in detail with mainly medical content and need about 30-45 minutes. This also shows that staff members of the higher service for health care and nursing make the time for a nursing consultation dependent on whether there are enough other colleagues in their shift, so that the everyday nursing activities are not neglected. Also, the inclusion in the doctor's consultation is decisive for the staff of the senior health and nursing service for the length of a nursing consultation. In the case of recurring conversations, it depends on whether the patients are ready for further information and whether a confidential and empathetic relationship has already been established in advance.

- **Space for the preparation and implementation**

The lack of opportunities to prepare the content and the patients for a nursing consultation in a suitable room in peace and quiet is also cited. Due to the presence of fellow patients and visitors in the multi-bed rooms, and the colleagues going in and out, it is not possible to implement a trusting and protected private sphere for a nursing consultation. This in turn makes it difficult to build an empathetic and genuine relationship between the participants.

4.2.4 The strategies for action

The strategies of action of the staff members of the higher service for health care and nursing in nursing counselling in the oncological setting yielded the following results in the study:

- **Fears of carers in the nursing counselling interview**

Fears are raised when talking about existential topics such as pain, suffering and death. Further insecurities of the staff members of the senior service for health and nursing care are triggered by questions which stem from the patients' and their relatives' knowledge of the internet. Fears are also raised when demanding relatives interrupt the nursing consultation with additional questions.

Rogers describes in his client-centred concept that positive appreciation, authenticity and unconditional acceptance are the basic variables of counselling. The basic attitude is characterised by empathic, non-possessive warmth, sympathy and acceptance (cf. Elzer/Sciborski, 2007: 84f).

- **Individuality of the carer in the nursing counselling interview**

This in turn leads to a situation where too much preparation by the nurses of a counselling session gives the impression that it is a lecture. In these situations, younger nurses seek contact with experienced colleagues so that they can review the discussion together before it begins and address any unplanned questions. This gives the nurses a certain amount of security beforehand. Experienced staff members design their counselling sessions individually, not only by answering questions, but also by adapting to the respective situation and recognising what the patients need at the moment:

"It always develops a bit differently, there are some where it's just enough.... A long conversation is almost too much (IP2: 139-142)".

- **Exchange in the team after a nursing counselling interview**

After the end of a difficult counselling session, there is a heightened exchange between the team colleagues, in which the counselling situation can be repeated and reflected upon. This kind of reflection helps the staff not to put too much pressure on themselves with their own high expectations. Expectations in nursing consultations are mainly based on the assumption that the prepared contents and main topics must all be addressed in the consultation so that they can have a positive feeling at the end of the discussion.

Communication is a circular exchange without a clear beginning or end. Cause and effect lie in the interpretation of the communication partners. Watzlawick assumes that we have our own reality and hold it to be true, and that this subjective reality determines our actions. This can lead to different understandings or misunderstandings in the communication relationship (cf. Watzlawick, 2016: 20).

- **Family relationship in a nursing counselling interview**

The staff members of the higher service for health care and nursing perceive the presence of relatives during the nursing consultation as unpleasant and stressful. Unexpected questions and interruptions by relatives during the conversation unsettle and irritate the nurses. This in turn leads to them becoming attached to the patients and thus excluding relatives. This one-sided relationship leads to conflicts in communication. The communication and interaction is decisive for the quality of the counselling provided by the staff of the senior health and nursing service.

Roger's theory of personhood causes self-healing and self-actualisation forces to be released between nurses, patients and their relatives. In relation to a conversation in the oncological setting, it is therefore particularly important that nurses create a climate of respect, authenticity and understanding so that these self-actualisation forces are activated and positively support the course of the disease of patients and their relatives. For a concept of nursing counselling in the oncological setting, it is therefore necessary that the individuality and subjective perspectives of the patients and their relatives are included (cf. Koch-Straube, 2008:24).

4.2.5 The consequences

The consequences in the nursing counselling interview of the staff of the higher service for health care and nursing show the following results:

- **Reflection and rituals**

All six nurses use the exchange with team colleagues before and after a nursing consultation. Reflecting on the content after a discussion helps to ensure that the staff members do not put themselves under too much pressure with their own high expectations. It also shows that five out of six nurses use rituals to relieve themselves after stressful discussions, such as taking deep breaths or shaking out their hands, but also the daily shower after duty helps to let go. Rituals support and challenge the resilience of nurses in the oncology setting.

- **Documentation**

A lack of and incomplete documentation of the nursing counselling talks is cited by three nurses as a complication of recurrent counselling.

Carers often do not perceive the activity of counselling as a continuous task. As a result, counselling activities are not documented and thus not regarded as professional care activities (cf. Huper/Hellige, 2007: 102).

- **Education, training and further education**

Although two of the nurses have completed further training in oncology nursing according to § 64, no preparations are made on how a conversation should begin, be set up or end, or what happens if a patient breaks off the conversation. Also, five out of six nurses state that they were taught communication for a maximum of one day during their training and that they only acquired their competences in practice.

Health counselling and communication for nurses is regulated in the Federal Act on Health and Nursing Professions in Austria. The nursing core competences in § 14 (1) and (2) include, in addition to the autonomous activity of nursing, theory- and concept-guided conversation and communication. Furthermore, the multiprofessional area of competence in § 16 (3) of the higher service for health care and nursing includes nursing expertise in health counselling. Hospice and palliative care in § 22b also include counselling and/or training of patients and their relatives in dealing with symptoms and forward planning to identify wishes and needs for the last phase of life (GuKG, version of 25.05.2019).

5 Summary and résumé

The perspective of the nurses, their reality and their experience during a nursing counselling interview with patients and their relatives in the oncological setting are in the foreground of this research work. The personal experiences of the staff members are subjective experiences from which insights for the nursing counselling interview in the oncological setting are gained. From the researcher's point of view, grounded theory is suitable for answering her research question, since it is about the process of experiencing a nursing counselling interview in the oncological setting and its difficulties. Six interviews were conducted with staff members of the senior service for health care and nursing in the oncological setting. The study took place in the direct research field of an oncology department in a primary care hospital in Vorarlberg. An open procedure and a narrative interview guide for data collection describe the inductive and theory-developing procedure of this research work. The selection of the test persons for this study was carried out in a process-accompanying manner. The researcher assumed that each case from the field of study would contribute something to the subject-related theory. She made sure that the interviews were transcribed and analysed in a timely manner. In this way, the resulting concepts for the further interviews were tested for their validity. This is in line with the theorising anchored in grounded theory. The researcher's field notes and observations of the subjects were included in the theory building. The aim of this study is to experience, identify and understand basic themes that come up in the context of a nursing counselling interview in an oncology setting, as well as difficulties, obstacles and the unexpected in the context of a counselling interview.

Based on the research question "How do staff members of the higher service for health care and nursing experience the nursing consultation with patients and their relatives in the oncological setting of a primary care hospital in Vorarlberg?

Coding paradigm (cf. chapter 4.2 Presentation of results). Coding paradigm)

Counselling is an integral part of care, which contributes to well-being and recovery. Help-oriented everyday conversations in professional care should not be confused with counselling, as this is carried out in a goal-oriented and methodically professional manner. Everyday counselling often takes place accidentally in everyday care and is carried out intuitively by the caregivers. Despite all this, counselling is still associated with informing, instructing and training. Interaction and communication is a central part of counselling. In expert counselling, specialised nurses provide their knowledge and experience. This takes place in the oncological setting between the patients, their relatives and the staff of the higher service for health care and nursing within the framework of a nursing counselling session in a primary care hospital in Vorarlberg. In this process counselling, the nurse sees him/herself as a supporter and supplicant of a pending development during the illness process. The counselling process is often dynamic, because the individual phases overlap, but also merge or repeat. This means that carers are in a position to respond directly to the difficulties encountered by the patient.

The initial conditions to be able to offer counselling include the ability to perceive patients and their relatives individually. The willingness to develop and use oneself to understand situations is another competence in counselling. The researcher's results show that the nurses distinguish between younger and older patients. This is because they assume that younger patients ask more and more detailed questions in the conversation, but also because the nurses identify more strongly with patients of the same age or younger. Furthermore, it can be seen that less experienced nurses invest more time in the preparation of a nursing interview, because they assume that their professional knowledge of the treatment plan and the course of the disease improves their competences in counselling and thus the quality of counselling. This means that the prerequisites for successful counselling in nursing must include knowledge of theoretical principles and methodological competence so that the counselling process can be designed in a goal-oriented and systematic way.

In order for nursing counselling to be carried out in an oncological setting, the framework conditions and the agreement between the participants are the prerequisite for a helping relationship to develop. The setting influences the quality and limits of a conversation. Institutional framework conditions restrict the carers in their counselling activities. The prerequisite for counselling is, among other things, sufficient time to get to know each other and openness. In everyday care, there is a lack of time, but also a lack of the right space. Multiple-bed rooms make it difficult to establish initial trusting contact with the patients. The necessary working conditions for shaping a counselling process must be supported by superiors. The time frame for the preparation and implementation of a nursing counselling interview in this study depends on several factors. The staff members of the higher service for health care and nursing distinguish whether it is an extensive first consultation and whether there are enough other colleagues on duty, and whether they were already able to be present at the doctor's clarification consultation. The contents and main topics are also decisive for the duration of a nursing consultation in the oncological setting. Furthermore, it can be seen that nurses with little or no professional experience invest more time in the preparation of a nursing consultation. Furthermore, the nurses complain that there is a lack of rooms for the preparation of a nursing counselling interview in which it is possible to prepare for the interview in peace and quiet.

The basic attitude of the counselling is characterised by empathic, non-possessive warmth, sympathy and acceptance. The action strategies of the staff members of the senior service in the nursing counselling interview showed that the nurses overcome fears, prepare themselves individually for the nursing counselling interview and have an animated exchange in the team before and after an interview. Fears are raised when the discussion deals with existential topics such as pain, suffering and death. Further uncertainties in the discussion arise from unprepared questions by the patients and their relatives, which are asked from incomplete and partly wrong internet research. Individual preparation for a nursing counselling interview differs in that younger colleagues prefer contact and exchange with experienced colleagues before an interview, so that they can prepare the planned interview together before it begins. This gives them a certain security and reinforces their competences. In contrast to this, it can be seen that experienced staff members of the higher service for health care and nursing make their conversations dependent on adapting to the respective situation and recognising what the patients need at the moment. After the end of a difficult nursing counselling session, there is an increased exchange among the team colleagues by repeating and reflecting on the discussion situation and contents. The presence of relatives during the counselling session is also perceived by the carers as unpleasant and stressful. This is because their unexpected questions and interruptions during the conversation unsettle and irritate the carers. This in turn leads to carers becoming attached to the patient and thus excluding relatives. Conflicts in communication with relatives arise from a one-sided relationship between the nurses and the patients, which excludes the relatives. The communication and interaction is therefore decisive for the quality of the counselling provided by the staff of the higher service for health care and nursing. For a concept of nursing counselling in the oncological setting, it is therefore necessary to include the individuality and subjective perspectives of the patients and their relatives.

The consequences of the staff members of the higher service for health care and nursing in nursing counselling showed that nurses reflect the content verbally with their colleagues before and after a difficult conversation, but that the conversation is insufficiently or not at all documented in writing. Nurses often do not perceive the activity of counselling as a continuous task. As a result, counselling is not documented and thus not perceived as a professional nursing activity. As helpful support after difficult nursing counselling sessions, nurses use rituals, such as deep breathing or shaking out hands. Rituals support and challenge the resilience of nurses in the oncology setting. Furthermore, it can be seen that the nurses have hardly received any theoretical knowledge in communication and nursing counselling during their training. This leads to the fact that they only acquire their competences in practice. Health counselling and communication for nurses is regulated in the Federal Law for Health and Nursing Professions in Austria. The nursing core competences include, among others, theory- and concept-guided interviewing and communication. Furthermore, the multi-professional area of competence includes nursing expertise in health counselling. This has the consequence that targeted education, further education and training as well as reflected professional practice are necessary for nurses to be able to fulfil their counselling function.

The results of this study show that communication in the form of counselling is performed with a high level of professionalism by nurses, but they lack awareness of their interactive work. Nursing counselling in the oncology setting is influenced by the nurses' attitude and understanding. This leads the researcher to the conclusion that the specific professionalism of interactive work must be demanded, and therefore further education and training in the nursing sector should be expanded. The results will be passed on to the nursing management so that appropriate measures can be initiated.

6 Outlook and Limitation

The development of a grounded theory is a very time-consuming undertaking that requires a high degree of self-structuring on the part of the researcher, despite the given methodological orientations. In this study, the researcher attempted to present the results in a transparent and comprehensible way by means of a detailed description of open and axial coding, the quotations from six interviews and with the help of a coding paradigm. Axial coding from the researcher's perspective was therefore sufficient for answering the research question. The results are determined by the researcher's interpretation and contain perceptions and events from the professional environment of the interview participants. As a ward manager and researcher in her own professional field, the author must assume that the senior staff withheld information, but also idealised their experiences. All interview participants spoke very openly about their experiences in the interview, but one interview participant stopped the conversation after a few minutes at her own request. Due to the limited time frame, the researcher conducted the interviews alone. Expanding the sample to include a clinical social worker in this study would have been another exciting aspect. This was because it had revealed interesting differences between professional clinical counselling and nursing counselling in the oncology setting. Involving patients and relatives would also have been another perspective in nursing counselling. A silent observation by the researcher during a nursing counselling session had led to additional results.

In connection with the central results mentioned above, it became apparent to the author that not all aspects have been investigated in sufficient depth. Among other things, the phenomenon of *"rituals before and after a stressful conversation"* emerged. This seems to have a high relevance for the caregivers' self-care and mental hygiene, because several interview statements revealed that they use different rituals during stressful conversations. Hand shaking, changing uniforms, showering after duty were mentioned, but also an intensive exchange with team colleagues was reported. Therefore, further studies on the use of rituals before and after stressful conversations of the nurses are of great interest. The question for further research is therefore: What is the significance of rituals in care?

Further findings for the researcher were that characteristics such as fears in dealing with existential questions and insecurity regarding their professional competences were especially expressed by younger nurses in the oncology setting in the nursing consultation. As a result, fewer and fewer young nurses wanted to work in an oncology department. This raises another interesting question for the future: What are the developments in the future of nursing and what measures are necessary for nurses to decide to work in the oncology setting?

It is also evident that the many years of professional experience of nurses in the oncology setting is a decisive characteristic for the quality of nursing counselling in this study. This in turn shows that older staff members have a wealth of experience that can be passed on to younger colleagues. From this it can be concluded that a special value should be placed on long-serving employees. As a result, another question arises for the author: How can older and experienced staff pass on their experience and knowledge in the oncology setting?

Another phenomenon that the researcher identifies in the study is that nurses observe a lack of communication and cooperation between nurses and doctors, which can lead to misunderstandings and conflicts between the professions. The lack of cooperation between doctors and nurses raises another question: How can interdisciplinary cooperation succeed in the oncological setting?

A final finding of this study is that nurses are increasingly confronted with new media in counselling. This means that patients and their relatives already come to a counselling session with a certain amount of prior knowledge, and this creates new challenges for the nurses, as there is an unmanageable flood of information on the internet. In this context, a final question arises for the author: What possibilities do new media offer in counselling for carers? What are the advantages and disadvantages of online counselling?

BIBLIOGRAPHY

BACHMANN-METTLER, Irene (2007): The future role of nurses in oncology. Der Onkologe 4: 356.

BAUMER, R. (2008). Counselling and communication. In: Baumer, R. & Maiwald, A. (2008). Oncological care. Stuttgart: Thieme, pp. 341 - 343.

BAUER, Nina, BLASIUS, Jorg (eds.) (2018): Handbuch Methoden der empirischen Sozialforschung. 2nd fully revised edition. Springer VS © Springer Fachmedien Wiesbaden GmbH, part of Springer Nature 2014,2019.

BGBl. 108/1997 as amended: Bundesgesetz uber Gesundheits- und Krankenpflegeberufe (Gesundheits- und Krankenpflegegesetz - GuKG). Online in the WWW at URL:
https://www.ris.bka.gv.at/GeltendeFassung.wxe?Abfrage=Bundesnormen&Gesetzes number=10011026 [Accessed 25 May 2019]

BOEHM, Andreas (1994): Grounded Theory - How Models and Theories are Made from Texts. In A. Boehm, A.Mengel, & T. Muhr (Eds.), Understanding Texts: Concepts, methods, tools (pp. 121-140). Konstanz: UVK Univ.-Verl. Konstanz. Online in the WWW at URL:
https://nbn-resolving.org/urn:nbn:de:0168-ssoar-14429 [Accessed 25 May 2019]

BREUER, Franz, DIERIS, Barbara, LETTAU, Antje (2009): Reflexive Grounded Theory. An introduction to research practice. VS Publishing House for
Social Sciences. GWV Fachverlage GmbH, Wiesbaden.

BREUER, Franz (2010): Reflexive Grounded Theory. An introduction for research practice. 2nd edition, VS: Wiesbaden.

FEDERAL MINISTRY of Labour, Social Affairs, Health and Consumer Protection (2019): Patientencharta und Rechtsgrundlagen. Online in WWW at URL: https://www.gesundheit.gv.at/gesundheitsleistungen/patientenrechte/inhalt [Accessed 23 May 2019].

CARSON, David, GILMORE Audrey, PERRY, Chad, GRONHAUG, Kjell (2001): Qualitative Marketing Research. London; Thousand Oaks; New Delhi: Sage Publications.

CHARMAZ, Kathy (2006): Constructing Grounded Theory. A Practical Guide Through Qualitative Analysis. London; Thousand Oaks; New Delhi: Sage Publications.

CORBIN, Juliet, STRAUSS, Anselm (2003): "Grounded Theory Research: Procedures, Canons, and Evaluative Criteria". In Interviewing: Volume IV, Nigel Fielding (ed.), London; Thousand Oaks; New Delhi: Sage Publications.

DEH-HINDENBERG, Andrea (2007): Patient needs in speech therapy. The quality of communication determines the evaluation of therapy. Forum Logopadie, 4: 26-33.

EKERT, Barbel, EKERT, Christiane (2010): Psychology in Nursing. 2nd revised edition. Georg Thieme Verlag KG. Stuttgart.

ENGEL, Roswitha (2006): Health counselling in nursing. Importing concepts and integrated training curriculum. Facultas, Vienna.

ENGEL, Frank; SICKENDIECK, Ursel (2005): Guidance - an independent field of action with new challenges. In: Pflege & Gesellschaft, 10th volume, No. 4, 2005:163-171.

ELZER, Matthias, SCIBORSKI, Claudia (2007): Communicative competences in nursing. Theory and practice of verbal and non-verbal interaction. 1st edition. Verlag Hans Huber, Hogrefe AG, Bern.

EZZY, Douglas (2002): Qualitative Analysis. Practice and Innovation. London: Routledge.

FLICK, Uwe (2007): Qualitative Social Research: An Introduction. 2nd ed. of the completely revised and expanded new edition. Reinbek: Rowohlt.

FROSE, Sonja (2010): Was Sie uber Beratung wissen sollten. Schlutersche Verlagsgesellschaft mbH & Co. KG. Hanover.

GuKG - Bundesgesetz uber Gesundheits- und Krankenpflegeberufe (2013): Gesundheits- und Krankenpflegegesetz in der Fassung BGBl. I Nr. 185/2013.
Online in the WWW at URL:
https://www.ris.bka.gv.at/GeltendeFassung.wxe?Abfrage=Bundesnormen&Gesetzes number=10011026 [Accessed on:25.05.19]

GITTLER-HEBESTREIT, Norbert (2006):   Care counselling in the
Discharge   management.   Basics-Content-Developments.   Schlutersche   Verlag, Hanover.

GLASER, Barney, G., STRAUSS, Anselm (1967): The Discovery of Grounded Theory. Strategies for Qualitative Research. London: Weidenfeld and Nicolson.

GLASER, Barney, G. (1978): Theoretical Sensitivity. Mill Valley, CA.

GUBA, Egon, G., LINCOLN, Yvonna, S. (1985): Naturalistic Inquiry. Newbury Park: Sage Publications.

HAUSMANN, Clemens (2014): Psychology and Communication for Nursing Professions. A handbook for training and practice. 3rd revised and expanded edition, Facultas Vienna.

HELFFERICH, Cornelia (2011): The quality of qualitative data. Manual für die Durchführung qualitativer Interviews. 4th edition, VS Verlag fur Sozialwissenschaften, Wiesbaden.

HOLLOWAY, Immy, WHEELER, Stephanie (2010): Qualitative Research in Nursing and Healthcare. 3rd edition, Wiley-Blackwell, West Sussex.

HUMMEL - GAATZ, Sonja, DOLL, Axel (2006): Unterststützung, Beratung und Anleitung in gesundheits- und pflegerelevanten Fragen fachkundig gewahrleisten, Urban & Fischer, Munchen.

HUPER, Christa; HELLIGE, Barbara (2007): Professional care counselling and health demands for the chronically ill. Framework - Basics - Concepts - Methods. Mabuse, Frankfurt am Main.

KENNEDY, Sheldon, L. (2005): Communication in oncology care. The effectiveness of skills training workshops for healthcare providers. In: Clinical Journal of Oncology Nursing, 9, 305-312. doi:10.1188/05.CJON.305-312.

KOCH-STRAUBE, Ursula (2008): Counselling in Care. Hans Huber Verlag, Bern.

KOCH-STRAUBE, Ursula (1997): Fremde Welt Pflegeheim. Bern.

KROHWINKEL, Monika (2007): Rehabilitative process care using the example Apoplexy patients. Demanding process care as a system. Hans Huber Verlag. 2nd edition, Bern.

KREDDIG, Nina, KARIMI, Zohra (2013): Psychology for Nursing and Health management. Psychology for professional practice. Wiesbaden: Springer Fachmedien.

LAMNEK, Siegfried; KRELL, Claudia (2016): Qualitative Social Research. Textbook. 6th revised edition. Beltz Verlag, Weinheim: Basel.

LANGKAFEL, Peter, LUDKE, Christian (2008): Breaking Bad News. The breaking of bad news in medicine. Heidelberg, Munchen, Landsberg, Berlin: Economica Verlag, Verlagsgruppe Huthig Jehle GmbH.

GUIDELINE PROGRAMME Oncology (German Cancer Society, German Cancer Aid, AWMF): Palliativmedizin für Patienten mit einer nicht heilbaren Krebserkrankung, Langversion 1.1, 2015, AWMF-Registernummer: 128/001OL. Online in the WWW at URL:
http://leitlinienprogramm-onkologie.de/Palliativmedizin.80.0.html
(access:05.05.2019).

LUEGER, Manfred (2009): "Grounded Theory", in Qualitative Marktforschung: Konzepte - Methoden- Analyse. Renate Buber and Hartmut H. Holzmuller (eds.),

Wiesbaden: Gabler.

MAIWALD, Andrea, WECHT, Daniel (2006): Modules desired. Oncology care in Germany. Padua 3: 14.

MARGULIES, Anita, KRONER, Thomas, GAISSER, Andrea, BACHMANN-METTLER, Irene (2011): Oncological Nursing. 5th ed. Springer-Verlag Berlin Heidelberg.

MEY, Gunther, MRUCK, Katja (eds.) (2011): Grounded Theory Reader. 2nd updated and extended edition. © VS Verlag fur Sozialwissenschaften | Springer Fachmedien Wiesbaden GmbH.

MEY, Gunter, MRUCK, Katja (2007): Grounded Theory Methodology - Remarks on a prominent research style. S. 11-42 In Gunter Mey & Katja Mruck (Eds.) *Grounded Theory Reader* Koln: Zentrum fur Historische Sozialforschung.

MUTZECK, Wolfgang (2008): Cooperative counselling. Fundamentals, Methods, Training, Effectiveness. 6th edition. Beltz Verlag, Weinheim, Basel.

NESTMANN, Frank (1997): Guidance as a resource requirement. In Nestmann F. (ed.): Guidance - Building Blocks for Interdisciplinary Science and Practice. Tubingen.

NESTMANN, Frank (1997): Big Sister is Inviting you - Counselling and Counselling Psychology. In Nestmann F. (ed.) op. cit.

OLK, Thomas (1989): Farewell to Experts. Social work on the way to an alternative professionalism. Juventa, Munich.

Osterreichische Krebshilfe (2018): Family members and cancer. Brochure of the Austrian Cancer Aid. Vienna.

RADZIEWICZ, Rosanne, BAILE, Walter, F. (2001): Communication skills. Breaking bad news in the clinical setting. Oncology Nursing Forum, 28: 951-953.

RIETMANN, Stephan, SAWATZKI, Maik (eds.) (2018): The future of guidance. From behavioural to relationship orientation. Social work as welfare production. Springer Fachmedien Wiesbaden GmbH.

ROGERS, R. Carl (1999): Non-directive counselling. 9th ed. Frankfurt am Main.

ROGERS, R. Carl, SCHMID, F. Peter (1991): Person-centred. Foundations of theory and practice. With an annotated counselling talk by Carl R. Rogers. Matthias-Grunewald-Verlag Mainz.

ROGERS, R. Carl (1972): Client-Centered Therapy. Houghton Mifflin Com., Boston

1942: Die klientenzentrierte Gesprachspsychotherapie, Kindler Verlag. Munchen 1972].

ROHNER, Jessica, SCHUTZ, Astrid (2012): Psychology of Communication. Basic knowledge in psychology. Springer VS Wiesbaden.

Sozialgesetzbuch (SGB) - Elftes Buch (XI) - Pflegeberatung. Online in WWW at URL: http://www.sozialgesetzbuch-sgb.de[Accessed 28 May 2019].

SCHAEFFER, Doris (2008): The first step towards recovery. On the difference between information, education and counselling. In: Padua, Vol. 3, Issue 2, pp. 6-11.

SCHAEFFER, Doris, MOERS, Martin (2008): Survival strategies - a phase model on the character of coping behaviour of chronically ill patients. In Care and Society. 13 (1): 6-31.

SCHWARZER, C., POSSE, N. (1986): Counselling. In B. Weidenmann & A. Krapp (Eds.), Padagogische Psychologie: 631- 666. Psychologie Verlags Union

STRAUSS, Anselm (1998): Fundamentals of Qualitative Social Research. Data analysis and theory building in empirical sociological research. Munich: Fink Verlag.

STRAUSS, Anselm L. (1987): Qualitative Analysis for Social Scientists. New York: Cambridge UniversityPress.

STRAUSS, Anselm; CORBIN, Juliet (1998). Basics of qualitative research: Techniques and procedures for developing grounded theory (2nd ed.). Thousand Oaks, CA, US: Sage Publications, Inc.

STRAUSS, Anselm, CORBIN, Juliet (1996): Grounded Theory: Fundamentals of Qualitative Social Research. 1st edition 1996. Translated from the American by Solveigh Niewiarra and Heiner Legewie. Psychology Publishers Union. Weinheim.

STRAUSS, Anselm; CORBIN, Juliet (1990): Basics of qualitative research: Grounded theory procedures and techniques. Newbury Park, Calif.: SAGE

CHUDIN, Verena (1990): Helping in Conversation. A guide for carers. Recom Verlag. Basel

WATZLAWICK, Paul (2016): You can't not communicate. The Reading Book. Compiled by Trude Trunk and with an afterword by Friedemann Schulz von Thun. 2nd, unchanged edition. Hogrefe Verlag. Bern.

WORLD HEALTH ORGANISATION/WHO/Europe(1980): Medium term Programme for Nursing and Midwifery in Europe (1976, 1983). Copenhagen.

WEYLAND, Peter (2013): Psychoonkologie - das Erstgesprach und die weitere Begleitung. With a foreword by Joachim Weis. Schattauer GmbH, Stuttgart.

WOLFSTETTER, Lothar (1984): The teachings of Xenon and their significance for psychagogy. In: Becker, Helmut et. Al. (Eds.): Michel Foucault, Freiheit und Selbstsorge. Materialis-Verlag, Frankfurt.

Future of Care (2018): FORUM2018^33:181-185 https://doi.org/10.1007/s12312-018-0415-2 Published online:4 April2018 ©Springer Medizin Verlag GmbH, part of Springer Nature 2018.

ANNEX

ANNEX 1

A narrative guideline interview with staff members of the higher service for health care and nursing in the oncological setting of a primary care hospital in Vorarlberg.

The oncological counselling interview - a field of tension in the oncological setting from the perspective of the staff of the higher service for health and nursing care

Date/Time   .2019 from to

Interview duration ___________________________

Interviewer Karola Muther

Interviewee ___________________________

Introduction

My name is Karola Muther. I am the ward manager of an oncology department in a primary care hospital in Vorarlberg. The study aims to show the challenges during a counselling interview in the oncological setting from the perspective of the staff of the higher service for health care and nursing.

The aim of my survey is to record the current situation in a primary care hospital in Vorarlberg so that supportive measures can be introduced in the future.

Annex 2

Declaration of consent and data protection declaration for the collection and Processing of personal interview data

91

Interviewer/researcher Karola Muther

Interview date/time

Interview location

Participation in this interview is voluntary and you have the option to cancel it at any time. This interview will be recorded on a tape recorder and then written down by the researcher Karola Muther. The scientific analysis of your data will be anonymous. All text passages that you do not wish to use will be removed. Personal data will be kept separate from interview data and will not be accessible to third parties.

I hereby declare that I agree to participate in this interview of my own free will. I agree to a tape recording during the interview and to anonymised data processing afterwards.

Name and signature of the interviewee(s)

Bludenz,

Appendix 3: Narrative guide for the interview

<table>
<tr><td>

Research question: How do staff members of the higher service for health care and nursing experience the counselling interview with patients and their relatives in the oncological setting in the regional hospital Bludenz?

Date:

Age:

Further training according to § 64: yes/no

Guiding question/incentive to pay:

Please describe to me how you feel in a counselling session with your oncology patients and their relatives? How do you experience the relationship between relatives and patients? What situations come to mind when you talk to patients and their relatives?

</td></tr>
</table>

Table 1: Survey instrument - guiding themes/research question (own representation)

Content aspects	Maintenance issues	Enquiries
Role of the carer: - Familiar - Associate - Competition Feelings of the Carer: - Fear/uncertainty - Distance/Nearness - Trust/	- What else can you describe when you think about your conversations and the respective situations? - Is there anything else from your point of view? - What happened next?	- How do you prepare for an interview? - What thoughts do you have before a conversation? - How doyoustart Talk? - How do you describe your Relationship to the Patients? - What role do you play during a conversation? - Which situations in the Do you find the conversation pleasant or unpleasant?
- Empathy Self-care of the Carer - Mindfulness - Acceptance Communication - verbal - nonverbal		- Which contents are particularly challenging for you? - How do you experience the relatives in conversation? - How is your relationship with the relatives? - What support can you imagine to make a conversation positive from your point of view? - How do you deal with emotions on the part of How do you deal with patients/friends? - How do you deal with your own emotions during a conversation? - How do you end a conversation? - What is the significance of such a conversation for you? - What role does a How do you use such a conversation in the care of patients and relatives? - How do you feel after the end of a Talks?

		- During your training, were you exposed to such Talks prepared?

94

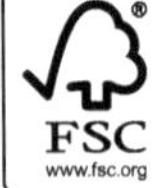

Printed by Books on Demand GmbH, Norderstedt / Germany